The Big Apple Diet

Dr. Alexander Matos

Celestial Arts
Millbrae, California

Celestial Arts
231 Adrian Road
Millbrae, California 94030

Cover and book design by Jill Losson
Illustrations by Colleen Forbes
Editing by Pathfinder Publishing Services
Typography by HMS Typography, Inc.
Printed by George Banta Company

First printing, February 1982
Manufactured in the United States of America

Library of Congress Cataloging in Publication Data

Matos, Alexander, Dr.
    The Big Apple diet.

        Includes index.
            1. Reducing diets.   2. Autogenic training.
3. Reducing diets—Recipes.
I Title.
RM222.2.M377   613.2′5   81-21559
ISBN 0-89087-339-9 (pbk.)   AACR2

1 2 3 4 5 6 7 8 9 10 — 88 87 86 85 84 83 82

Dedicated to the overweight people who have suffered the slings and arrows of their thin counterparts.

Special thanks to my loving wife and best friend, Bernice, and to
my sweet daughters, Caryn and Debra, for supporting me
through it all. Thanks also to, my agent, Mary Jane Ross,
for believing in me and, finally, a great big
"Thank You" to my patients who made this book possible.

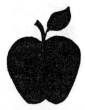

Preface

My own body led me to the truth about successful dieting. For years, as a doctor, I tried to help people lose weight by using traditional dietary methods such as calorie counting. I even tried a not-so-traditional method, hypnosis, but nothing seemed to work. Many of the patients lost weight, but the loss was always temporary.

At the time, I tipped the scales at 250 pounds. I was a good 100 pounds overweight. When a patient occasionally looked me in the eye and asked why I was so fat, I felt embarrassed and resorted to a limp and unsatisfactory, "Do as I say, not as I do."

One winter night I was returning home after working late at the office, pleasurably anticipating a little snack—waffles and vanilla ice cream sounded just right. I was disappointed to find that the delicatessen—the only store open at that hour—had only pistachio ice cream, a flavor I detested, but I bought a quart anyway. As I was approaching home, I decided to take just a little taste in the hope that I would like it after all. I tore off a corner of the carton and used it as a scoop. The first taste was terrible, but, in the hope that the next mouthful might be better, I had another. I still disliked the taste, but not enough to stop myself from walking into the kitchen and devouring the entire quart within five minutes.

That was my moment of truth. I had stuffed myself with food I did not even like. My stomach was swollen against my belt. The whole situation was insane. I determined, then and there, to find the most effective way to take and keep weight off, for myself and for others.

So, out of frustration, the Big Apple diet concept was born. You see, I'm a native New Yorker—born and bred in the Big Apple—and I developed my ideas with the help of my fellow Big Applers—my patients.

As used in this volume, the terms **thin, slender,** and **trim** have the same meaning. And the words **overweight, fat,** and **obese** are synonymous, as well.

A **thin person** is one who is satisfied with his or her weight and does not desire to lose. An **overweight person** is one who is not satisfied with his or her weight and does want to lose. For example, if you tip the scale at 150 pounds and are satisfied with that weight, you would be thin (and probably would not be reading this book). If you weigh 150 pounds and desire to lose, however, you would be fat. Being fat or thin is purely an individual or subjective state; it is the way you see yourself.

Food means any substance, solid or liquid, that contains calories, and which one puts in the mouth and swallows. The terms **eating** and **drinking** will also, therefore, be used synonymously.

Contents

CHAPTER ONE
Surviving in a Thin World

Historically, overweight people have been underdogs in Western society. To be considered attractive, a man or woman is almost always thin or, at the very least, not fat.

In earlier times, as today, overweight has been the target of ridicule. Lord Chesterfield disdainfully remarked that, "obesity and stupidity are such companions that they are considered synonymous." St. Jerome observed that, "a fat paunch never breeds fine thoughts." Literature is full of such comments.

Modern times have not changed society's attitude. Often enough, there is actual discrimination. Statistics show that those seeking employment frequently lose out, even though studies have long since established that there is no relationship between weight and intelligence or between weight and the capacity to perform on most jobs. A recent study of executives earning over fifty thousand dollars a year pointed out that over 90 percent had slim, trim bodies. Not long ago social workers representing the state of Wisconsin ruled that Gordon and Barbara Ray, happily married and having met all other criteria, could not adopt a child because they were overweight. It was only out-raged public protest that made the state back down from its arbitrary position.

The very fact that many people regard an obese body with emotions ranging from humor to disgust cannot fail to affect a fat person's psyche. Clearly re-flected in other people's eyes is exactly what they think, and the realization of second-class status, inferi-ority, and difference hurts.

Nor is there any escape. Life in the modern world is too interdependent for one to allow oneself to be-come isolated from everyday encounters, much as one might like to. Nevertheless, many overweight people suffer from a sense of isolation in a variety of ways. They are conscious of being objects of scrutiny and often derision if they join organized activities. When they dance, swim, play softball, exercise, or stand nude in a locker room or shower, they are acutely self-conscious. They know that they are being looked at and, in a sense, judged.

Even those who overcome embarrassment know that they are different. If someone observing them takes their excess weight matter-of-factly, they inter-pret it as an obvious attempt to make them feel less like freaks than they really feel themselves to be. And sometimes it is harder to live with pity than with ridicule.

Sexuality

Self-awareness in the bedroom is also significant. Dread of how one must appear to one's partner can affect sexual pleasure, performance, and even desire.

Fat people suffer on a more subtle sexual level as well. There is a strong sensual element in the pleasure that thin people obtain from being attractive. I call it **secondary sexuality.** In our society, we obtain the greater part of our sexual gratification indirectly. Primary sexual expression (physical sex) simply is not readily available because of social and moral codes or even simple convenience. However, secondary sexuality is always possible—and even likely.

There are, for example, those pleasures to be had in the games men and women play all the time. People thrive on using their sexuality to derive pleasure in this way. It is harmless, fun, and has nothing to do with sexual promiscuity. Nor does it mean that slim types enjoy sex more than fat ones. It simply means that they gain more pleasure from being physically attractive and give pleasure in return—far more than they could gain or give from the solitary pleasure of overeating.

The overweight must work much harder to obtain a slice of this secondary sexual pie, usually by being clever and witty, which is the stereotype of the jolly fat person. Sometimes power—monetary wealth and position—helps such a person to be "attractive." But it takes a lot of something very special to get even a small slice with which to compete on any level other than physical attractiveness. Does that sound unfair? Well, it is. Should people be taught to think of themselves as misfits if they do not enjoy listening to Beethoven or watching a football game? Of course not. And yet society, overtly and covertly, demands that all be thin. Since overweight people are a part of society, they must conform in order to be maximally content. To put it another way, being thin offers more pleasure than overeating.

Carrying excess weight is like going through life with a dull headache. The discomfort is not enough to incapacitate you or send you to the hospital. Friends are not aware of your suffering. But your body makes your life miserable. Recognition of the way you feel should help spur you on to get rid of that "dull headache" by never forgetting the basic message:

You must develop a willingness to substitute the deep pleasure of being as attractive as possible for the temporary pleasure of food.

Short-Term versus Permanent Weight Loss

Once they realize that by becoming thin they can enjoy more of life's pleasures, many people make a foolish mistake. They become enthusiastic and take off weight as a short-term goal. They fail to understand the concept of becoming thin as a permanent condition. Many patients have told me that they wanted to lose weight to "get married," or to "meet a man (woman)." This is probably one of the worst reasons for an overweight person to attempt to lose weight because it is a temporary reason for a specific and limited purpose.

In the course of a day, I see many newly divorced and separated people. They listen attentively and largely "agree" with what I have to say. Most make good patients and lose weight beautifully. But is their reason for losing rooted in a genuine desire to be attractive, or are they simply doing it in order to find a new mate? Experience has taught me that once a specific goal is achieved—for example, losing weight to find a mate—the fat person becomes satisfied, and the desperation that fired the determination to lose weight disappears. The old ways resurface along with the fat. Even when the goal of finding a new mate is not achieved, many get discouraged—"There's no one out there for me anyway"—and they promptly regain lost weight.

Dozens of people desperately shed body fat for weddings or other social functions, but the weight goes right back on when the affair is over. Even "I want to be thin so I'll look good in a bathing suit," is a poor reason because it is temporary. When summer is over and cool weather arrives, the motive is gone. Remember, your reason must be permanent if it is to be effective.

Beating the Genetic Blues

The argument has long been waged over whether many of society's social and psychological ills are caused by genetic (inherited) or environmental factors. In truth, both share responsibility for the heavy person's plight.

Genetic influence

Are people born with the tendency to overeat? To determine the answer, psychologists performed a simple experiment with great success. They tested fat and thin people to learn if there was a difference in their ability to identify the taste of certain foods. They used twenty common foods such as lamb chops, fruits, nuts, vegetables, and the like, ground to the consistency of baby food. The foods had no relationship to their original form except for the taste. Without exception, the fat people recognized all of the foods. Nearly all of the thin people were totally confused.

The conclusion is that fat people have a keener sense of taste than thin people. This suggests that such a person derives more intense pleasure from food and would, therefore, be likely to attach more importance to it. Of course, it is impossible to measure mathematically the pleasure derived from eating. We have all, however, witnessed the gusto with which the overweight person devours a meal in comparison to the enthusiasm shown by a thin table partner. The fact that one is more sensitive to taste makes it harder to stay away from food, and this sensitivity is apparently a genetic factor. An individual with one overweight parent stands a 40 percent chance of being overweight. One with two stands a whopping 80 percent chance of being overweight, whereas a person with neither parent overweight stands only a 20 percent chance of gaining weight.

Studies have shown that certain strains of animals tend to gain weight more quickly than others. For example, Angus cattle eat more and are a heavier breed than Jersey cattle. The same is true of certain hogs, which naturally eat more and thus fatten more quickly. Genetics as a causative factor in obesity cannot be disputed. Do not, however, become discouraged because of the genetic factor. Unlike the color of our skin, which is 100 percent genetically determined, eating is totally voluntary; we can control and change our eating habits. I repeat: **you** can control and change your eating habits; **you** can substitute the pleasure of being more attractive for the pleasure of eating.

Environmental influences

Environment also plays an important role in "forming" the fat person. In many ethnic groups, starchy, sweet foods seem to be the rule rather than the exception. There is growing awareness of nutritional values, but if you are over sixteen years old, it is more than likely that much damage has already been done. Even television can be a fattening influence. Not only does TV invite laziness (the average family's set is turned on for about six hours a day), but we are also brainwashed by it!

Statistics have revealed that the average American child sees twenty thousand television commercials by the age of eleven and that at least 50 percent of those commercials promote foods loaded with sugar. Many nutritionists call sugar the "killer carbohydrate."

There has also been a proliferation of junk foods, that is, foods that are sweet to the taste, high in empty calories, and low in nutritional value. Manufacturers (major food-processing companies), spend millions of dollars every year on advertising and public relations. To advertise their products, they use models with healthy, tanned skin and gleaming white teeth. Yet the junk food some of these manufacturers produce is both harmful and fattening. Relatively low in cost, it is designed to snare the attention and the appetites of today's active children and young adults, who are always on the run and often eat whatever is handy to grab on the way to school, the movies, or a ball game. Bad eating habits inculcated and reinforced by years of unfortunate television advertising are hard to break. All the blame cannot be placed on food processors. If people refused to buy junk food, if they turned away from oversweetened, fattening, and nutritionless foods, food manufacturers would stop providing them.

Thus, both genetic and environmental factors influence our eating habits and affect our physical state. Both can be counteracted by consciously focusing on the underlying objective of substituting the **permanent** pleasure of being thin and more attractive for the **temporary** pleasure of food. Thus, the rest of this book will be devoted to teaching you exactly how to attain that goal.

CHAPTER TWO

The Road to Thin

There are four types of thin people. Three are naturally or genetically thin, which means that the eating
tendencies are inherited from parents. The first of the
genetically thin types, Type I, simply does not have
much appetite for food. You can always spot such
people in a restaurant. They never touch bread,
always leave part of the main course, and toy with
dessert. Although they may claim to enjoy eating,
food has never been really important to them. Their
trim bodies are a gift of nature rather than a testi-
mony to efforts at self-improvement. Entertainer
Johnny Carson typifies this naturally thin type. In
talking with fat guests on several television shows, he
has assured them that "I eat as much as I want, and I
never get fat." In truth, Mr. Carson does not know
what eating "much" really means. He simply has
never had a large appetite.

The second genetically thin type is the most devious. The person publicly "eats like a horse and never seems to put on weight. Envied and hated by the overweight society because of this seemingly mystical ability, Type II people, in truth, have no special magic. They are simply high-energy, physically active people who literally "burn" fat because they are hyperactive.

The third type of genetically thin person, Type III, like the second type, overeats in public. The secret is that, in private, the person does not eat much at all. Walter, one of my first patients and a favorite (I do have favorites), is a good example. Walter was thin and in no way had a weight problem. Since I had plenty of free time, as most professionals do in the beginning, Walter and I would sit for hours and rap about everything from his problem to space exploration. One evening Walter, who knew I had a weight problem, tantalized me with the following story: "I just had the greatest malted milk shake I ever had in my life! They made it with two Mello Rolls, and it was delicious!"

Remember Mello Rolls? They were devilish, cylindrical-shaped portions of delicious ice cream, and Walter's description of the "great malted" made my mouth water. Walter was my last patient, and he left shortly before the dinner hour. I remarked, "I bet you can hardly wait to get home and have dinner." He stared at me in amazement and said, "Doc, I'm stuffed to the gills. That malted **was** my dinner. I couldn't eat another bite tonight." I shook my head in surprise, knowing that, if I had consumed that malted, it would not have stopped me from having a full meal. I realized that Walter was one of many thin people who seem to eat a lot, but they really do not.

It is the fourth type of thin person, **controlled** thin, that concerns us. These people are thin by design. They have the tendency to get fat, but refuse to succumb to the temptation. Type IV people tend to enjoy food, to eat a lot, and to become fat, but their eating is controlled, the appetite is tempered, and the individual remains slender. The remainder of this book is devoted to understanding this type of thin person.

The Way to Being Type IV

Great truths are simple. **Thin people obtain more pleasure from being thin than from eating excessive food.** The key is the word "pleasure." The pleasure a thin person feels in being thin is directly related to a larger truth that we all know. I had just never applied it to dieting. Certainly we all recognize that the search for pleasure is one of the most potent of human drives. There are many ways in which we seek pleasure: accumulating money, seeking social acceptance or sexual fulfillment, having and enjoying children, reading, personal hobbies, sports—the list is endless. Physically, the body has numerous pleasure zones. One of the most important is the mouth. The mouth speaks, laughs, cries, makes love, and is even used for breathing when the sinuses are blocked. And, of course, we eat with our mouths.

To the overweight, eating is the summit of all pleasurable experiences: tasting a favorite food, chewing
it, and swallowing are pure joy.

On occasion I would ask a patient, "If by magic I
were to create your favorite foods and desserts and
snacks so that they were as delicious as usual, but
completely nonfattening, would you choose the food
or sex with your spouse?" The answer in most cases
was, a giggle, a smile, and a choice: the food.

In terms of pleasure, food has at least six
advantages:

1. **Food is close at hand.** You may enjoy
   playing tennis, but you have to go to a tennis
   court to participate. Food is as close as the
   cookie jar.
2. **Food is available at any hour.** If you enjoy
   going to the theater, you are limited as to
   when and where productions are staged. But
   the light in the refrigerator is always on when
   you open the door.
3. **Food is relatively inexpensive.** If you love
   high-speed sports cars, you must have the
   money to afford one. But, in our society, people of all economic levels can afford some
   kind of food.
4. **Food can be enjoyed alone.** If you want to
   play tennis or dance, you need a partner. You
   can enjoy food by yourself.
5. **Food is socially acceptable.** Sex is highly
   pleasurable, but must be experienced in

private. No one objects, however, to your eating a bag of potato chips or a candy bar in public.

6. **Food provides instant pleasure.** Playing the piano well is pleasurable, but learning to play takes time and effort. When you put a spoonful of ice cream in your mouth, your gratification is immediate.

The Rationalization Detour

Faced with a situation that we would rather not accept, we rationalize. Rationalizations are simply excuses. A person who has been fired for incompetence rarely admits to personal failings, but finds excuses: "My boss didn't like me"; "The foreman had it in for me." The student who fails a subject often complains that it was not presented properly or that there was no time to study.

Rather than admit that they choose to overeat and thus to be overweight, people soothe their consciences with excuses. I have heard them all, many, many times, and you will surely recognize them. The most common one usually comes out as: "I just don't have enough willpower." A person using this convenient excuse implies the lack or loss of an innate human capacity (willpower) that others, that is, thin people, were born with. Consequently, overeating is not the fault of the overweight rationalizer, who has neatly ducked the burden of responsibility by placing it on some inherited or genetic factor.

What that clever person lacks is motivation, not willpower. Motivation—a deeply inspired purposefulness—creates the necessary thrust to accomplish a goal. It is instructive to see how rapidly such a person develops the willpower to diet when there has been a separation or a divorce and he or she must get thin to win another mate. Cigarette smokers also complain about lack of willpower. The willpower miraculously appears when they learn they have a heart defect or cancer. Such examples indicate that motivation, not willpower, governs action.

It is also helpful to understand the difference between voluntary and involuntary control. One woman who came to me was deeply depressed, and a hundred pounds over her normal weight. She complained that she "lacked dietary control," even though her lack of control made her miserable socially and personally. I was able to help her by explaining that the beating of her heart is an involuntary action that cannot be controlled but that eating is voluntary and **can** be controlled. Voluntary means that she and she alone decides when and what to eat. She was ultimately able to acknowledge the falsity of her argument, and it was this recognition that gave her the necessary understanding to follow my reducing program. She lost the excess weight with no further trouble.

Then there are "life's vicissitudes," which are beautiful rationalizations that provide a hundred or more excuses, all blamable on the heavy burden of daily living. People say they overeat because they are bored, unhappy, irritated, lonely, unloved, anxious, angry, nervous, depressed. Upon closer questioning, however, they also admit to overeating at happy times such as weddings, social gatherings, and vacations. The emotional conditions listed are normal enough. All of us, thin or fat, experience them. To say that you can diet successfully only when you are completely happy is ridiculous; negative emotional states are as much a part of life as are excitement and happiness. Fat people who are being honest with themselves will admit that they eat under **all** emotional conditions—happy and miserable.

Reference to life's vicissitudes is especially popular among overweight homemakers. The nonworking group complains of confinement to the kitchen and constant proximity to food as reasons for not staying on a diet, while working homemakers complain that dining out makes it difficult to diet. Overweight people must learn to become thin within the framework of their existence.

An exotic rationalization popular among the more sophisticated overweight group attributes overeating to psychological trauma. Some common expressions are: "I overeat because if I get thin I'll have to face the world, I'll have to go out and compete." "I'm convinced I have a death wish and am using food as a weapon with which to kill myself gradually." "Somewhere in my past I underwent a deep emotional trauma." "My mother always used food as a reward, or withheld it as punishment." "I'm punishing myself for the guilt feelings I've had because my father and I weren't on good terms when he died." "I've failed in every way—personally, sexually, financially—and food is the only thing that never lets me down." "As a child my parents forced me to overeat because people were starving overseas." I could go on and on.

I admit that there is a small group of overweight people—from talking to psychologists, I would estimate that they represent less than 2 percent of the total—who have true psychological impairments. Such people are so deeply troubled that they exhibit many symptoms of disturbed behavior, and excess weight is but one small manifestation of their problems. Most of those who use psychological trauma (self-diagnosed or diagnosed by well-meaning but misinformed psychotherapists) as the reason for overeating, use it as an excuse to do what they really want to do—overeat.

An interesting case involves a woman whom we shall call Susan. Her seven-year-old daughter was struck by a car and killed. Susan took the death very hard, and, within a year, she had gained forty pounds. Therapists who were trying to help her adjust to her loss agreed that she was compensating for her daughter's death by overeating. During our initial consultation, however, I learned that Susan had always been predisposed to overeating and, as a teenager, had constantly been on a diet. As genuinely upset as she was over the death of her child, she was also using it as an excuse to do what she had really wanted to do, which was to eat more than she should. Susan was shocked by such an apparently unfeeling accusation, but she was honest enough to think about it seriously. When she gave up using the tragedy as an excuse to overeat, she had no difficulty losing the forty pounds.

The myth about compulsive eating deserves special attention. When an individual claims to be a compulsive eater, there are similarities to the person who excuses overeating by saying that he lacks will-power. There is the implication, in both instances, that the person has no control over eating processes. This is not true. If you were to offer a compulsive eater a fee of one million dollars with the stipulation that he or she adhere to a diet, the "compulsion" would probably disappear, as if by magic. People who justify obesity by claiming to be compulsive eaters are simply attempting to shirk responsibility for their actions. They are only kidding themselves; people know exactly what they are doing when they eat.

Another phrase that has a good scientific ring to it is "metabolic dysfunction." It is referred to in a variety of ways: "My metabolism is slow or poor." "I really eat very little." "I smell food and get fat."

By such statements, fat people infer that because of endocrine (glandular) malfunction, either acquired or inherited, their ability to utilize or "burn" food is impaired. The thyroid gland is most often blamed. Patients tell me they "think" an underactive or sluggish thyroid (hypothyroidism) is responsible for their condition. Again, there are some fat people, about one in a thousand, who suffer from true metabolic dysfunction. Even with hormonal correction (addition of thyroid extract), such patients remain overweight.

In a study of this problem, the Mayo Clinic concluded that the incidence of obesity due to thyroid disease is minute. A wise person once said: "The only gland at fault in obesity is the salivary gland." Rationalizations are comforting, but they do not change the fact that in most cases three factors alone determine whether a healthy person gains or loses weight. They are food intake, energy output, and body surface area.

Trading Away Excess Weight

Once overweight people admit to the fallacy of rationalizing, they must be willing to trade the pleasure obtained from consuming excess food for something that will offer more pleasure. There is a difference between trading or exchanging something and giving it up or having it taken from you. It is one thing to trade ten thousand dollars for a new automobile and quite another to have the money stolen from you at gunpoint. Fat people must think of dieting as trading the pleasure of overeating for another, more intense pleasure, rather than as giving up the pleasure of eating. This requires an effective reason to eat less and, thus, become thin.

Reasons to Make the Journey

There are many reasons to be thin. Most are logical and sound. Below are some of the more popular ones that overweight people use, as well as reasons why they **do not** work.

For my health. If an overweight patient comes to my office complaining of back pain, my first words are: "Lose weight." Most health practitioners agree that excessive weight creates or aggravates a surprising number of human ills.

In the United States our biggest health problem, cardiovascular disease, is often associated with overweight. Fat people are also more susceptible to diabetes, arthritis, high blood pressure, diseases of the kidney, and gall bladder attacks, as well as liver and back problems. Even cancer has recently been linked to obesity.

Most health practitioners agree that the constant physical exertion of carrying a fat body has a life-shortening effect, and yet the threat to health seems to be the weakest motivation to lose weight. We do not seem to care enough about our health. Notice, I did not say that we do not **care**; I said that we do not care **enough.**

The only time health seems to be an effective reason for losing weight is when a problem is current or acute. Even then, the concern seems to be temporary. When the health emergency is over, the weight is usually regained. How many times has a person who just suffered a coronary lost many pounds only to regain them upon feeling better? Theoretically, health is an excellent reason for losing weight. Pragmatically, it does not work.

For my husband or wife. Many people say they would like to lose weight to please their mates. Ironically, the reverse seems to hold true. Once people commit themselves to one another, the pressure is off. Most of us are conditioned to stay as attractive as possible in order to meet a likely partner, fall in love, get married, and raise families. Unfortunately, people with a tendency to gain weight feel secure after marriage, and the floodgates open.

A spouse's affection can also act as a deterrent to losing weight. Many testify that the spouse has said, during the course of an attempted diet, "Oh, you can have one little bite." Or, "You're doing just fine." Or, "Eat today and start tomorrow."

In reality, every spouse harbors conflicting feelings about a mate's losing weight. A common fantasy is exhibiting the newly attractive thin spouse, thus arousing the envy of friends. But the mate who becomes thinner and more attractive is likely to attract more attention, and that calls for being on guard more often. When a person complains about a mate's excess weight, it may be only lip service paid to the ideal of being thin—an ideal that might be upsetting if it were actually achieved.

For my children. This handy reason implies any one or a combination of three things: (a) they want to set a "good example" for their children to follow, (b) they want the children to be proud of their trim parents, or (c) they want to be healthier and thus live longer for their children.

Although these reasons are sound and logical, they do not work either. Most parents know that children tend to follow their example, and yet these same parents, who would probably defend their children with their lives, will not stop overdrinking, or quit smoking, or lose weight. Mr. Jones, a six-foot, three-hundred-pound man, disagreed with me. He and his wife were both overweight. Both of his sons were thin and extremely weight conscious. He believed that his and his wife's weight problem alerted the children and helped keep them thin. He even added that the boys were constantly badgering their parents to lose weight. Mr. Jones was kidding himself. His children were not thin because of him, but in spite of him.

If parents are beer drinkers, it does not mean that **all** their children will drink beer. It means that the chances of the children drinking beer will be greatly increased. It is the same with obesity. A negative example does not encourage positive results. And children who badger their parents to lose weight are usually concerned with the health hazards associated with obesity.

For myself. This is by far the most popular reason for becoming thin, but it does not work either. **Everything** we do is for ourselves, including eating. We overeat (and thus become fat) for our own pleasure. Imagine yourself abandoned on a desert island where food is plentiful. It would never occur to you to go on a diet, and yet you would be there by yourself.

For you to say that you are going to lose weight for yourself is like saying that, "water is wet." The statement is true enough, but it does not help you lose weight.

The Destination

We have already established that thin people derive more pleasure from being thin than from eating to excess. I needed to know more—the exact nature of the pleasure they obtained, and why they stayed thin. In order to find out more, I devised the questionnaire that appears in Chapter 12. Not only did I ask the questions of my own overweight patients, but I also queried slim patients and friends.

The first reaction by the thin groups was that they enjoyed wearing attractive clothes. Still, people don't dress up to sit around by themselves. For whom do they want to be attractive? For others, of course. **Thin people get and stay thin because they enjoy being physically attractive.** Their goal is mainly to please people whom they do not know or even hope to know, and perhaps might not even want to know. Thin people pamper their bodies with flattering clothes and exploit their attractiveness in all their contacts with others.

Some call the wish to be maximally attractive simple vanity. Others call it pride or self-esteem. Overweight people do not possess enough of it. This does not mean that fat people are not attractive. Many are well groomed and dress tastefully. It means that they lack the desire to be **maximally** attractive.

For fat people to become thin, they must learn to **think** like thin people. They must think of dieting as trading, rather than giving up, one pleasure (overeating) for the more intense pleasure of being more attractive. With a different mental attitude, dieting no longer means deprivation, unhappiness, suffering, and temporary sacrifice.

Social relationships with one's own sex are involved as well. Many thin people of the same sex are in competition with one another. This "competitive sport" acts as companion motivation for the thin person to remain thin. In case you had not noticed, today's executives take pride in staying slim.

Turn to the questionnaire in Chapter 12 to discover your own attitude toward dieting. Answer each question honestly. This exercise will enable you to compare your thinking, your developed responses toward eating, with those of people who have succeeded in becoming and staying slim. The resulting profile will provide the basis on which you can apply the principles discussed throughout this book.

CHAPTER THREE
The Truth About Dieting

The chances are that you have probably tried to lose weight and have had difficulty doing it. You may have gone on all kinds of diets, but none worked, that is, really worked. You might have lost some weight, but promptly regained it.

Why Most Diets Fail

Many people who have failed to diet successfully were misinformed or confused, or both, to begin with. They accepted the traditional concept of dieting as a negative rather than a positive act, a depressing, uphill battle against powerfully ingrained eating habits. Without realizing it, they started out expecting to be defeated.

But did they really have a chance? Every diet in history has been aimed at reducing food intake, which is good. But the problem with most diets is that they accent food. They emphasize eating rather than the self-knowledge that leads to control over one's appetite.

Overweight people by the thousands have come to me in despair over diets that have not worked, or have worked only temporarily. They have gone on high-protein diets, low-carbohydrate diets, water diets, milk diets, banana diets, grapefruit diets, chemically balanced diets, health food diets—even fasts—hoping to slim their bodies. Many have finally been driven to taking barbiturates, amphetamines, and hormones.

Many diets would be laughable, if only they did not inflict so much misery and result in so great a waste of effort and emotion. For example, one diet, which advocates "filling up" with unlimited low-calorie foods such as broccoli or celery, simply makes fat people yearn for the **real** stuff, such as ice cream and cake. Another advises a half a cup of spaghetti. I've never met a fat person who can be satisfied with a half a cup of spaghetti.

All such diets fail to recognize one basic and vital fact. No diet that attempts to placate appetite by limiting or substituting foods can satisfy a person on a lifetime basis.

Only a dietary education that looks beyond food to physical and emotional factors will enable a dieter to undertake an eating program that takes fat off and keeps it off. Today, the average overweight American is as fat as ever, if not fatter, which testifies to the failure of the many reducing systems offered to the

American public. When New York's Yankee Stadium was rebuilt recently, there were nine thousand fewer seats in the same area. Does this indicate that the average American is becoming fatter?

Motivation in Dieting

Successful dieting is more a matter of correct thinking than one of painfully restricting eating. This does not mean that correct thinking replaces control over eating and drinking. Both, of course, are required. The purpose of this book is to show how one leads to the other.

I have been helping people lose weight for a long time, and, what is equally important, helping them to keep it off. Diet alone will not do it. Motivated diet will. Learning how to motivate yourself is not difficult; it can even be pleasant. And the results are well worth the effort.

As a doctor, I have worked for over twenty-five years with people who wanted to lose weight. Seeing them succeed has been a great pleasure, but what of the thousands of unsuccessful dieters who spend months, even years, suffering unnecessarily. They flounder, agonize, feel guilty—and remain fat. Instead of losing weight, they lose self-esteem, they are depressed, they are frustrated, they are defensive: "I'm overweight—so what? I like to eat. Is that a sin?"

They can succeed. They need a knowledge of the basic emotional and psychological factors that are the foundation of any effective eating regimen and the ability to control, rather than to be controlled by, those factors. Without this knowledge and ability, they waste time, money, and emotion and all to often simply give up: "What's the use? Nothing works. I'm overweight and that's how it is."

To diet is not merely to control the amount and the kind of food you eat. The problem is to learn how to stick to it. I believe that I can show you how to do it and how to have the body you want. The mental and physical factors that underlie successful dieting are positive. They are easy enough to understand. And they work.

Three Truths That Ensure Success

There are three truths that the overweight person must acknowledge in order to understand and cope with the problem:

1. **They eat consciously and voluntarily.** Fat people are always aware of what they eat. Occasionally they try to fool themselves by quickly swallowing a couple of cookies while talking on the telephone, claiming to be "preoccupied" and not fully conscious of their actions. But they know exactly what they are doing. Nobody ever picks up a gun and forces food into their mouths.

2. **They anticipate or obtain pleasure from eating.** This is the toughest admission of all for overweight people to make, but it is a hard fact. Even though they may not be hungry;

even though they dislike what they are eating; even though they feel guilty before, during, and after the act of eating; even if they have a severe head cold and cannot taste the food—they still eat. This is because fat people are driven as much or even more by **anticipatory** pleasure than by the actual food they consume. The mental picture of eating is the first act of a two-act drama. It triggers the actual face-stuffing that follows. Why do they do it? Because the prospect of **some** pleasure is better than **none**. This was my greatest weakness.

3. **They are overweight because they overeat.**
   This is the most important of the three truths. Overweight people must understand that they are fat primarily because they eat too much food. Remember, food—steak, potato chips, alcoholic beverages, or whatever—is any substance that contains calories. If you eat enough of any food, even though low in calories, you will gain weight.

One of my patients, a woman in her forties, was a very cooperative patient and lost weight steadily for several weeks. But then her weight loss slowed and finally stopped, even though she swore that she was not deviating from her diet. After a long doctor-patient discussion, she finally revealed that she was eating great quantities of fruit. When I told her that this was her problem, she said in genuine surprise, "Why doctor, I never knew fresh fruit was fattening. I thought I could eat as much fruit as I wanted." Once she gave up eating the excess fruit, she started losing weight again. Parenthetically, such people always say "fresh" fruit—presumably distinct from canned, cooked, or frozen—as if being fresh removes the calories.

The path to successful dieting will be clear when an overweight person can look in the mirror and say honestly:

I eat consciously and voluntarily;
I anticipate and obtain pleasure from eating;
I am overweight because I overeat

Be aware that these three admissions are very difficult to make, because any person making them is accepting the responsibility for being overweight, admitting that he or she makes a conscious choice to overeat and to be fat. True, such people would like to be thin in much the same way that many of us would like to be rich and famous, but they are not about to make the effort to achieve the desired ends. When it comes right down to it, the fat person chooses the pleasure of food over the pleasure of being thin. It is that simple, but this fact is hard to recognize and accept.

Criteria for a Successful Diet

One point should be established early: the Big Apple Diet is not punitive; it does not require willpower, self-denial, or physical discomfort. Instead, it is based on the conviction that no diet can work if people must struggle desperately to stay on it. Every overweight person is a complex being with many physical and mental attributes, and my program is designed to let each dieter realize his or her own potential.

Devising a diet to help overweight people shed weight and keep it off required, first, an eating program that made sense nutritionally. A second consideration was whether it could be practical and pleasing. Here are eight criteria a successful diet should meet:

1. You do not feel hungry.
2. You do not have to use willpower.
3. You take no pills or drugs.
4. You can dine out at most restaurants.
5. You can adjust the diet to fit your needs.
6. Nobody needs to know you are dieting.
7. You do not have to count calories.
8. You do not have to weigh most foods.

The system described in this book is designed to help you lose the desired amount of weight and keep it off. Over the past fifteen years, I have treated more than three thousand patients with weight problems. Most had tried other diets, fashionable or faddish, from steak for breakfast to total fasting. All of the diets claimed miraculous results. The dieters invested great energy and emotion—and considerable suffering—only to discover that the age of miracles seemed to have passed. It has not. Such patients are now happier, thinner people, who realize that they have done more than change the shape of their bodies. They have gained pride and purpose. They have found new satisfaction with themselves, their mates, their friends, their work. From being merely food-oriented, they have finally become free, emotionally as well as physically.

CHAPTER FOUR
Questions and Answers about Dieting

Misinformation and misconceptions about dieting are common. I have been asked the same questions again and again during my years of working as a diet counselor. In this chapter, let me list those most commonly asked.

Is there anything wrong with having a final eating binge before starting my diet?

There is **everything** wrong with such an orgy. True, there is a tradition for this sort of thing. The "bachelor party," for example, precedes the "giving up" of a man's freedom and acceptance of the responsibilities of marriage. The same theme is present in the "last dinner" of the condemned man, the prisoner about to be executed, who is given anything he wants to eat.

For the would-be dieter, wanting to have a final eating binge is a psychological mistake: acceptance of the fact that you are having a final moment of freedom before surrendering something of value. It is an admission that the diet you are about to embark on is a thing of horror, against which you are steeling yourself by cramming your belly full for one last time. In other words, you do not really want to diet. Your diet must be approached as a liberating experience, and your mind's eye must remain on the ultimate goal: a slimmer, more svelte you, a person who has gained mental mastery over eating instead of being mastered by it. The only thing you are about to give up is the displeasure of excess body weight.

How rapidly should I eat?

People who are overweight are generally faster eaters because they eat with intensity. Thin people generally eat more slowly, and anyone on a diet can profit by following their example. Eating slowly helps in two specific ways, both of which are psychological:

1. The pleasure of eating is extended over a greater period of time; therefore, the mental satisfaction lasts longer. As a result, there is less temptation to search for something additional to ingest at the end of a meal.

2. Eating slowly gives the feeling that you have control over your appetite and that you are in charge of yourself. This engenders a subtle feeling of "winning," of having made tangible progress in the effort to lose excess weight.

In addition, there is a practical reason for eating more slowly; one automatically chews more, thereby aiding the digestive system and general health by sending the food to the stomach in a more pulverized form. This makes the stomach's work that much easier.

Do protein foods burn up fat?

Sorry, but **no**. There is a factor in the bodily assimilation of sugar, fats, and proteins that is known as the Specific Dynamic Action of foods, commonly referred to as SDA. Briefly, it means that the body requires a certain amount of energy to break down and assimilate these foods. Proteins require more internal body energy (calories) to be absorbed than do fats or sweets. This means that, ounce for ounce, you can eat more proteins than fats and sweets and gain less weight. The amount of calories saved is rather small, however, and unlimited ingestion of proteins will result in obesity.

Can I lose inches and not pounds?

Generally speaking, losing inches (body measurements) and pounds go together. On occasion, however, there is a "shifting" of body fluids (mostly water) from one area of the body to another that may account for the phenomenon. Such "shifting" is at best temporary, very small, and difficult to measure. Overweight people who zealously measure their body parts every day and find such "shrinkage," seize on the fact to proclaim that, even though they have not lost weight, they have lost inches. They are kidding themselves.

Alma was a warm and intelligent lady who had a weight problem most of her adult life. Like most overweight people, she had been through the mill, having tried many methods of losing weight. She finally heard of a diet doctor who promised that, even if you did not lose weight, your body would shrink and you would lose inches. This idea appealed to Alma. She stayed with the "inch doctor" for two months, but remained at the same approximate weight level. Her husband did not notice any change for the better, although she claimed that she was losing inches. The situation began to cause great friction between them, and, during the third month of trying to lose inches, Alma was referred to me. I remember the case well; it is most rare for a husband **and** wife to consult me because of the wife's desire to be thin.

During the interview, I felt like a referee at a fight. Without taking either side, I persuaded Alma to try a different approach to losing weight. She became one of my most successful patients. Not only did she lose inches, but considerable weight as well. But I shall never forget something the husband sarcastically said during our first meeting: "You know, Doctor, if what she says is true, I'm going to have the only wife with a size six waist who weighs two-hundred pounds."

The only honest approach is to ignore the business about the inches and measure your progress by weight alone. This is a pure, or mathematically certain, measurement. I can promise that concentration on losing pounds automatically means losing inches.

How can I help my children stay (or become) thin?

Most people feel terribly guilty about producing children who are overweight. But it is not their fault, as statistics prove. If one parent is heavy, the chances are 40 percent that their child will be heavy too. If both parents are heavy, the odds increase to 80 percent. If both parents are thin, the chance is only 20 percent that a child will be overweight. As to influencing your children, the best attitude a parent can take is to refrain from berating the child and making him feel unloved, guilty, or unattractive. Do not scold a child if you see him overeat. The parent can succeed only by example: showing the child dietary self-control and exhibiting a strong desire to become or stay thin. Children automatically copy their parents. Do not encourage your child to finish what is on his plate because "millions of people are starving in India." When entertaining children, throw a party with active games. Hire a magician or a puppeteer, but do not make the highlight of the day a big feast. Again, your example is the most important factor. Even if you are overweight, the very fact that you are becoming thin will help your child want to become thin.

Isn't it a good idea to bring my own diet food if I'm invited out to dinner?

No. Absolutely not. In the first place, it is an insult to the host or hostess who has labored to prepare a fine meal. But beyond plain manners, this self-conscious act on the part of the person implicity says, "Look at me. Admire my marvelous self-control." Such a person may sit down at the dinner table and whip out a piece of chicken or a hard-boiled egg and really believe he is trying to be a good girl or boy. But the truth of the matter is that he's hogging the spotlight forcing everyone to make him and the diet at least a temporary center of attention. You must face the fact that occasionally social situations arise that are beyond your control. Simply make the best of it. Eat what is available in small amounts, selecting less caloric foods such as salad and vegetables.

Does toasting bread lower calories?

Sorry, no. But toasting does make it taste better. In whole wheat or enriched bread there is a slight loss of Vitamin B, but the loss is so little that it should not deter you from eating toasted bread.

Does washing vegetables, potatoes, and rice lower calories?

It makes the foods nice and clean, but that is about all.

Does margarine have fewer calories than butter?

Regular margarine has about the same number of calories as butter. However, diet margarine has only about half as many calories.

Does grapefruit cut fat?

The only thing grapefruit may cut into is your budget.

Is fasting the best way to lose weight rapidly?

No. It is the best way to guarantee that you will gain back whatever you lose. This subject is discussed fully in Chapter Seven.

Does losing weight make one weak?

I read of a case where a man and his wife were shipwrecked on an island and had to exist on nuts, berries, herbs, and grasses. Their intake was about a third as much as their normal diet. They both experienced weakness for about a week and were quite concerned that they were seriously ill. Then the weakness stopped. Incidentally, upon returning to civilization, the couple learned that they were both in better health than they had been previously. They also learned that they could exist in perfect health, and at a more satisfactory body weight, on 50 percent of the food they had ingested before they were shipwrecked and forced to "return to nature."

Can I overcome a weakness for a certain food by eating so much of it that I get sick?

No way. This subject was covered in Chapter Eight, but I have come across the situation so many times that I am adding a few words here. If, say, your weakness is chocolate, you will hate the sight of it for perhaps twenty-four hours, maybe for as long as seventy-two hours. But then you will be just as hungry for chocolate, and you will feel depressed because your eating binge not only did you no good, but it caused you to break your dietary routine for no good purpose.

Does my stomach shrink when I diet?

No. The popular belief that stomachs shrink when dieting is incorrect. X rays have shown that both thin and fat people have stomachs that have no relationship to their waist size. Appetite is **not** regulated by the size of one's stomach.

Is drinking water with meals helpful?

Water is OK before or after meals, but not during. This is because water tends to revive the taste buds and thus create a desire to overeat. Also, using water to wash down food dilutes digestive juices in the mouth and in the stomach and forces half-chewed food to be swallowed. This is not only bad for the digestive process, but it decreases the time that one spends eating. Remember that the more slowly one eats, the more satisfying it is.

Does smoking aid in losing weight?

Here is another myth that I will now put to rest. It is commonly believed that if you "keep your mouth busy" by smoking you will be less likely to be tempted to overeat. It does not work for the same reason that stuffing yourself with low-calorie foods such as celery does not work.

The overweight appetite cannot be placated by any substitute for the real thing. Smoking simply adds a new problem with which one will eventually have to cope. Just as many fat people smoke as thin people.

If I decide to go on The Pill (contraceptive) while I am dieting, should I expect to gain weight?

Yes. One of the ingredients of the pill is the hormone estrogen. It tends to inhibit the body's ability to excrete fluids. Thus, even though you are dieting, you may not lose weight immediately. After an adjustment period of a week or two, however, you will lose at the normal rate. Incidentally, if, while dieting, you discontinue using the pill, you probably will be pleasantly surprised because the water that you gained while taking it will be lost and your weight will drop dramatically.

Do vitamins stimulate appetite? Are they fattening?

The answer is **no** to both questions. Vitamins cannot stimulate a healthy appetite, and there is no appetite more healthy than that possessed by an overweight person. They can, however, help a thin person who has a poor appetite due to malnutrition. The average vitamin pill has about one calorie.

How do I deal with constipation?

When starting a diet, it is not unusual to experience a temporary change in the frequency of elimination, simply because your body is not receiving as much food as before. After three to seven days, however, the regularity of your bowel movement should automatically be reinstated. If it is not, then do the following:

1. Before each meal drink two glasses of water.
2. For your evening snack, substitute 3 prunes, plus

the juice from the preparation of the prunes, instead of your evening fruit. Prepare the prunes by boiling a glass of water and then placing the prunes in the boiled water in a closed container. When the prunes become saturated and soft, they are ready for eating.

3. Have any bran cereal for your morning meal. Follow this regimen for one week. When the problem is corrected, you may discontinue the dietary change. (Incidentally, after a period of constipation a bowel movement can weigh up to two pounds. This is no cause for alarm.)

Why don't I "feel" thin, even after I lose weight?

Because it takes time to change the image that the average overweight person has lived with for most of his or her life. I remember that, as a youngster, I was extremely overweight. Children, because of their immaturity, are often cruel. I was known as "Four-Eyes Fatso," because I also wore eyeglasses. Although it has been sixteen years since I shed my weight, I still tend to turn around, if, when I am walking down a street, a child yells, "Hey, Fatso," to another child. I remember those days. I should. I still feel their effects.

How do I handle night eating, due to insomnia?

A small percentage of people are middle-of-the-night eaters. The common complaint is that, because they have insomnia, they wander around their home and eventually end up at the refrigerator. After the dietary indiscretion, they feel better (but guilty) and find it easy to return to bed and sleep.

A simple psychological explanation will make the matter clear. Most overweight people insist that they cannot help waking up hungry in the middle of the night. In nearly all cases, however, these night eaters sleep soundly and do not awaken from hunger pangs while on vacation in hotel or motel rooms. Why? Simply because food is not available at these hours in such places. Overweight middle-of-the-night eaters must realize that they have developed the habit of mentally creating the insomnia to rationalize overeating. To eliminte this problem, you must use determination and the motivational principles explained in this volume. Make up your mind not to give in to the urge for one week. If you awaken during the night, remain in bed. This act will teach your subconscious mind that you mean business.

Isn't being socially active a way to keep from overeating?

Yes, within reason. Friends you really enjoy give you less time to think about what is in the refrigerator. If you are in love, the excitement of the romance—the happy times and experience shared—also serves to keep the interest in food to a minimum. Any form of social activity is legitimate, as long as you enjoy it. But you cannot go out with everyone you meet or join clubs and group activities simply to avoid eating. Any genuinely enjoyable social activity is helpful, but your frustration in not finding true enjoyment will inevitably turn you back to the satisfaction of food.

With diet pills can you eat all you want without gaining?

No. When amphetamines were legal, they were used extensively to curb appetite. I considered them dangerous, for I found that, without exception, they caused a standard pattern of behavior: the pills seemed to help for a while. Then they lost their effectiveness as appetite suppressants, and people began to eat just as much as before. In addition, many became addicted to the amphetamines. Not only did they still eat a lot, but they then had a drug problem as well.

Is it a good idea to start your diet with another person or persons?

No. Remember, all overweight people subconsciously compete with one another. More often than not, partners will be jealous if you lose and they do not. Also, if the others fail at their diets, they tend to "drag you down" emotionally with them.

Is it a good idea to enlist the aid of a spouse or friends to "police" you?

No. For many reasons, such as:

1. Others do not really believe that "this time" you are going to diet successfully, simply because you have "cried wolf" too often.
2. Dieting and dieters are usually boring to other people, who are concerned with their own problems.
3. Strange as it may seem, very few people actually

want you to be thin, especially those of the same sex. As long as you are fat, you are not a competitive threat; you cannot compete socially, athletically, or sexually.

So do not enlist the aid of another person. When dieting, be your own best friend.

Does dieting cause bad breath (halitosis)?

Bad breath most often occurs if there is a coexisting pathological condition of the oral cavity or the digestive system. It is also produced when the diet does not include foods that have to be well chewed, such as green vegetables. Such foods are called fiber. Grandma called them roughage. These foods tend to "clean" the teeth of deposits of other foods that might ordinarily be left to decay and thus create bad breath. Many fad diets do not provide enough fiber, but, in the diet given here, there should be no problem.

Is it a good idea to purchase tight-fitting clothes, to help me stick to my diet?

Let me answer this question with one of my favorite stories. In my fat days, it was impossible for me to find suits to fit my rather unorthodox shape (5'-5" with a 42 waist and 46 jacket). If I attempted to buy a suit "off the rack," by the time it was altered to fit I could have had it custom made. In addition, the altered suits never fit well. I decided to purchase custom-made suits. After I purchased my first suit, the tailor had my basic measurements and, on subsequent visits to his shop for additional suits, it was not necessary for him to remeasure me. I once visited his shop to buy a new suit, however, and told him to make the pants and jacket smaller because I was going to diet and lose weight. The tailor nodded his head in agreement. But when I came back to pick up the suit, I had not lost the weight and happily discovered that he had not made the clothes tighter as I had requested. When I asked him why, he answered, "Almost everyone asks me to make their clothes tighter, but experience has taught me to ignore them because they never take off the weight." This story has a clear moral. Do not buy tight clothes for **expected** weight loss. Do use and alter your present clothes until it is absolutely necessary to buy others. (I did so with a pair of trousers until the back pockets met.) Another factor is that buying clothes when you are halfway to your goal weight can act as a deterrent to losing all of the weight, for the new clothes will make you more attractive and may provide too much temporary happiness, tempting you to stop dieting. The answer is to buy only those clothes that are absolutely necessary until you complete your weight goal.

Will drinking plenty of water help reduce your appetite?

Water will never buffer the fat person's appetite. Appetite can never be destroyed because of non-caloric fillers, because appetite (as I have pointed out numerous times) is in your head, not in your stomach. Water, however, is important for the body to function properly, especially the elimination system.

When my stomach "grumbles," does that mean it's empty and needs food?

Nonsense. Grumbling stomachs are not complaining or empty stomachs. The noises coming from your intestines are caused by various foods and by enzymes that work during the digestive process. They have nothing to do with "time to eat."

CHAPTER FIVE
Eating and Dieting Effortlessly

Earlier I said that successful dieting stems primarily, if not exclusively, from correct thinking, and that the goal is to substitute the pleasure of being more attractive for the pleasure of excess food. Now, how do we go about it?

Wanting to change the way we think and act is not enough. We need help. The psychological tool we require is right at hand: Hypnosis II. With it, you will be able to stick to the diet, lose weight, keep it off, and change your thinking in the process. The effort will be simple and painless, and, by the time you reach your goal weight, correct thinking will be automatic and yours for life. Your diet and suggested menus are covered in this chapter, and Hypnosis II is the subject of Chapter Six.

How to Custom Design Your Diet

In looking over the food choices that follow, you will see that I have divided them into three groups, based upon desired goal weights. This is because we all have different food needs.

I once sat at the training table of a professional football team and watched a 225-pound linebacker devour four steaks so huge that the average person would not have been able to finish even one. After that, he had a tremendous salad and dessert. Every ounce of his body was trim and hard. He ate enormous quantities of food because he burned up a tremendous amount of body energy by physically exerting himself to near-exhaustion.

I also knew an Indian religious figure, a quiet, gentle soul, who spent the greater portion of his days sitting in silent meditation. At least four days a week, he imbibed nothing more than a single glass of milk. Slender, even skinny, he was still healthy and well fed. Because he was small and expended virtually no physical energy all day long, he needed scarcely any food.

Although the reader of this book is probably neither a professional football player nor a frail religious figure, these examples of extreme dietary behavior do illustrate how activity or occupation relate to the amount one eats. Other factors to be considered in the formulation of a reducing diet are age, height, sex, and body frame. Tall, large-framed people, for example, can eat more than their short, small-framed counterparts. Preadolescents, teenagers, and the elderly require professional supervision.

I purposely have avoided calorie or gram (carbohydrate) counting, for in the "long-haul" this method does not work. Most people who are overweight could probably write their own book about the calorie or gram value of foods.

Starting the Easy Way

Start by weighing yourself—with indoor clothing—sans shoes. For some people this is a traumatic experience, but it is necessary in order to evaluate future progress. Jot it down on the "Beginning Weight" line of the "Profit with Loss" Statement (Illustration 1) indicating the date and time in the appropriate space.

Weigh and record your weight **once a week**—always on the same scale, at the same time of day, and dressed in a similar way. Weighing yourself more often can be both misleading and harmful because we all lose weight at different times for different reasons. If a person is active he will sweat and lose water; if he is inactive he will gain water. This is particularly true of women who gain weight through water retention during their menstrual cycle. Daily weighings show fluctuations that are not accurate as a measure of true progress. Another danger of constant weighings is that a person who loses weight after a period of activity becomes overconfident and tends either consciously or unconsciously to celebrate. This celebration usually takes the form of eating.

Profit with Loss Statement

Goal Weight _____

Week	Weigh Date	Weigh Time	Weight	Previous Weight	Weight Change
Beginning					
1					
2					
3					
4					
5					
6					
7					
8					
9					
10					
11					
12					
13					
14					
15					
16					
17					
18					
19					
20					

Illustration 1

Be sure that you do **not** weigh yourself naked because naked is not your "true" weight. It is not the you that goes through the day wearing clothes that weigh anywhere from one to three pounds. Standing naked on a scale is "cheating," for, by eliminating those pounds, you tend to accept your lower weight, thereby increasing the temptation to eat more.

Establishing a Proper Weight Goal

Now it is time to determine the goal weight that you will achieve. The Weight Chart (Illustration 2) reflects what I consider proper weights, based upon my professional experience, for most people. For females eighteen to twenty-five years of age, subtract one pound for each year under twenty-five. Height as well as weight is measured without shoes.

In establishing a weight goal, one should pick the lowest possible figure. Most overweight people choose goals that are twenty to forty pounds over those of their thin counterparts. When I suggest that they attempt a lower weight, I receive two standard replies: The first is that, "I was never that weight in my entire life," to which I reply, "If I gave you a million dollars, would you refuse it based on the fact that you never had so much money before?" The second reply is that, "I was born heavier than that weight." By "born," fat people mean that, since they were never thin, it is impossible to become so now. This is not true.

There are reasons to aim for a super-thin weight level. If workers are told to quit at 5 o'clock, they begin to let down or get tired at 4 o'clock. If the next

Weight Chart

WOMEN (plus or minus 1 to 5 pounds)		MEN (plus or minus 1 to 10 pounds)	
4'-10"	97	5'-2"	130
4'-11"	101	5'-3"	135
5'-0"	105	5'-4"	140
5'-1"	109	5'-5"	145
5'-2"	112	5'-6"	150
5'-3"	115	5'-7"	154
5'-4"	119	5'-8"	158
5'-5"	123	5'-9"	161
5'-6"	130	5'-10"	165
5'-7"	135	5'-11"	168
5'-8"	139	6'-0"	174
5'-9"	143	6'-1"	179
5'-10"	146	6'-2"	183
5'-11"	150	6'-3"	187
6'-0"	153	6'-4"	192

Illustration 2

day the boss tells them to work until 6 o'clock, they zip by the hour of 4 o'clock and probably begin to tire at 5 o'clock. If you project your goal at twenty pounds higher than it should be, you'll probably get tired and lose enthusiasm forty pounds away from your true weight level. I see this happen all the time.

So project a very low weight. Even if you do not reach it, you will be thinner than you ever were before.

I believe that most overweight people really do want to be super-thin, but they are afraid to admit it because of past failures. Here is a psychological test to prove my point. Look at the "magic blackboard" (Illustration 3). It has weight levels, in increments of five, from 90 to 210 pounds. Place your finger on any number and that weight level will magically be yours forever—no matter how much you eat! Unfortu-

The Magic Blackboard

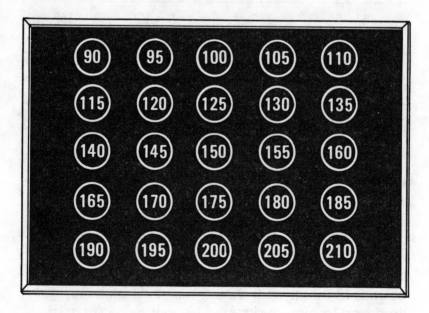

Illustration 3

nately this miracle cannot happen, but it does help to determine a psychologically sound weight goal. Incidentally, once you have chosen your magic number, subtract three pounds as a safety margin against temporary fluctuation, and write this figure on the goal weight line of the Profit with Loss Statement.

Having arrived at the figure, we can digress for a moment. In the days when I was seventy-five pounds overweight, I used to have lunch at a local diner that offered a different blue plate special each day. Nick, the owner and counterman, was a wonder. Not only could he be in a hundred places at the same time and still talk to all his regular customers, he also had a magnificent memory and never got an order mixed up. He knew exactly what dish went where. To observe him darting back and forth rapidly and unfailingly was a show in itself. Nick always identified his customers with the foods they ordered. As we'd sit at the counter talking, he would mumble, "Here comes the tuna on rye," or "Here comes the BLT down."

By talking to Nick, I learned that approximately 40 percent of his customers ordered the same foods day after day. That interested me. I could not understand how people could eat so monotonously. Weren't they bored? Because I was curious, I began studying these people and found that, without exception, they were all thin.

Then I began to study another group, which Nick called the "blue plate specials." They were people, like myself, who studied the menu for several minutes, mentally salivating over the choices, and then, more often than not, ordered the blue plate special. It was always good, the portions were plentiful, and it always included a heaping order of a house specialty, hash-browned potatoes. The "blue plate specials" were almost always overweight.

Apparently thin people did not spend much time thinking about what they wanted to eat. They wanted to finish the meal and return to whatever other activity engaged them. Overweight people fantasized about the choices on the menu as an initial step toward obtaining maximum pleasure from the eating experience. This fantasizing encouraged the tendency to overeat. The conclusion was obvious: **Sticking to the same food choices every day would probably keep an overweight person from fantasizing and, consequently, from overeating.**

That principle, which I have since had occasion to test exhaustively, has been adopted in my diet plan, which has three basic rules:
1. Stick to the same foods
2. Eat three meals a day. Do not skip, rearrange, or compensate. The three meals are breakfast (any time you arise after your major sleeping period), lunch (four to five hours after breakfast), and dinner (six to nine hours after lunch).
3. Do not eat between meals, except for drinking water.

It is possible to follow the diet easily and without thought. Use your thinking time for more important matters. But remember that the diet requires motivation to keep on working. That is why Hypnosis II, which will be discussed in detail in the next chapter, is as much a part of the diet as the list of foods. It is sufficient, here, to believe that you will be able to follow the diet and that you will succeed. My experience with both the diet and Hypnosis II over the past twenty-five years fully justifies that confidence. The diet menu appears in Illustration 4, (see page 56) and a more detailed discussion of it, including the quantities of foods allowed, follows.

Foods Permitted

The Big Apple Diet is nutritionally balanced with the proper amounts of proteins, fats, carbohydrates, vitamins, and minerals. Since vitamin and mineral requirements vary from person to person, however, I suggest beginning each day with a vitality cocktail for nutritional insurance.

Vitality Cocktail—To make a cocktail, mix a good vitamin-mineral supplement with four ounces of tomato or unsweetened grapefruit juice or eight ounces of water (I recommend water). Read the label to make sure that the vitamin-mineral supplement contains the recommended daily allowance (RDA) of all important vitamins and minerals. If the RDA is **not** defined on the label, do not purchase the supplement. You must also choose between a natural or a synthetic vitamin. Most authorities tell us that there is no difference between the two, but the synthetic vitamin contains certain inert additives (coatings, flavorings, and colorings). I prefer the natural form.

Illustration 4
Big Apple Diet Menu

Important Note: If you are pregnant or have a health problem or are
15 percent or more above your goal weight, see a physician before
starting this or any reducing diet.

BREAKFAST
Vitality Cocktail (see page 55)

One of the following groups:
Cheese—Bread—Margarine—Beverage
or
Egg—Bread—Margarine—Beverage
or
Cereal—Milk—Beverage
or
Yogurt—Beverage
or
Muffin or Bagel—Margarine—Beverage

LUNCH
One of the following groups:
Fish—Bread—Margarine—Lettuce Salad—Dressing
Beverage

---

or
Cheese—Bread—Margarine—Lettuce Salad
Beverage
or
Egg—Bread—Margarine—Lettuce Salad—Dressing
Beverage
or
Muffin or Bagel—Margarine—Beverage

DINNER

Soup (optional) or Wine (conditional)
Chicken—Vegetable
Mixed Salad—Beverage

BEFORE RETIRING

Fruit—Beverage (optional)

For Goal Weights between 90 and 150 Pounds

BREAKFAST

Cheese—Use hard cheese like Swiss, Muenster, American, mozzarella, or Swiss Gruyere. If possible, purchase packages containing individual slices that are approximately one ounce each (see unit theory on page 94). Avoid soft cheeses such as cottage, farmer, or pot cheese, as they are too strongly associated with past diets that have failed.

Egg—Either fry or scramble with a half teaspoon of diet margarin, or hard boil. Do not attempt to save calories by eliminating the margarine or by using a teflon coated pan. Greaseless cooking tends to make the egg rubbery, tasteless, and to appear less volu- minous. Never soft boil or poach, as eggs cooked by those methods are apt to be consumed too quickly.

LUNCH

Fish—Use tuna or salmon only, in the individual 3¾-ounce can (water packed if available; if not, regular, drained). Add lemon juice or ½ teaspoon of mayonnaise or eat plain.

Cereal—Any dry or wet cereal that can be purchased as individual servings, with a half glass (four ounces) of skimmed milk.

Yogurt—One container (eight ounces) of plain. Use extracts (vanilla, almond, etc.) to flavor the yogurt.

Muffin or Bagel—Bran (recommended), corn or English muffin, or bagel. These are "emergency" foods and should not be eaten too regularly. They are excellent when you are in a restaurant and find it difficult to obtain other selections. Another advantage to this occasional choice is that friends and well-wishers will not realize that you are on a diet. What diet includes a bran muffin? This prevents them from bending your ear about their own ideas of dieting or trying to discourage you.

Bread—One presliced piece of enriched white, rye, whole wheat, or protein bread, toasted or plain. Do not use diet, low-calorie, or thin-sliced breads. Eating such breads makes you rationalize that you can eat more and can lead to an eating binge.

Spreads, for bread, muffin, or bagel—Use ½ teaspoon of diet or half-calorie margarine. If not available (when dining out), use a small amount of butter or regular margarine.

Beverage—A cup of coffee, regular or decaffeinated, with a teaspoon of **whole** milk, or a cup of tea with lemon or a teaspoon of **whole** milk, or a glass of diet soda, or soda water. Learn to have your coffee or tea unsweetened (it really tastes better). If that is impossible, however, use an artificial sweetener or one level teaspoon of sugar per cup. You can choose between hot coffee and tea or iced coffee and tea. Hot beverages are recommended as it requires more time to consume them.

Lettuce Salad—One-quarter of an average-sized head of lettuce with dressing.

Salad Dressing—Dress salads with vinegar (wine or plain), salt and pepper, or a tablespoon of diet (low-calorie) dressing. The vinegar dressing is preferred as it is universally obtainable. Avoid overusing salt as it has a tendency to promote water retention.

Seasonings, Condiments, Herbs, and Spices—can be used according to taste on all foods in the Big Apple Diet. This includes catsup, mustard, and soy sauce.

DINNER

Soup (optional)—Clear soups, like chicken, beef, or onion. Avoid using dry bouillon cubes (past diets again). Homemade and restaurant soups are fine as long as they are clear.

Wine (conditional)—For occasional use only, such as a dinner out or special occasions. Choose a white wine (Chablis, or Moselle, perhaps, or rosé). Avoid sweet or sparkling wines (champagne) and all other alcoholic beverages including beer.

One further note: If you choose to have wine with dinner, be careful. Alcohol, even in small quantities, has the tendency to uninhibit. This "mental freedom" may encourage overeating. Be aware of the fact.

Chicken—From a quarter to half of a two-pound chicken. Those who choose the quarter lose faster. Do not bread or fry, but otherwise prepare as desired (with or without the skin), using condiments, spices, and herbs. Discard the skin before eating. All parts of the chicken are acceptable, including the dark meat. Fresh chicken is preferable, but frozen is permitted. Purchasing your favorite chicken parts is fine. Chicken cutlets, chicken rolls, and canned chickens are not recommended as they are eaten too rapidly.

It's better to have to contend with the bones because they require you to eat more carefully, therefore more slowly, and slower eating creates a more satisfied feeling. For more information on chicken, and some chicken recipes, see Chapter Thirteen.

Eat chicken for one month only. During the second month, alternate chicken with fish. From the third month on, alternate chicken and fish with veal. Do this until your weight goal has been achieved.

Fish (conditional, see page 66)—Eight ounces of pike, fillet of sole, red snapper, haddock, halibut, flounder, swordfish or whitefish. Do not bread or fry, but otherwise prepare as desired using condiments, spices, and herbs.

Shellfish—Six ounces of shrimp, scallops, or crab meat. Broiled only. One pound whole lobster, broiled or boiled without butter.

Veal (conditional, see page 66)—Six ounces of veal or a veal chop. Do not bread or fry, but otherwise prepare as desired using condiments, spices, and herbs.

Vegetable—One cup of cooked (fresh, frozen or canned) string beans, asparagus, bean sprouts, wax beans, broccoli, cabbage, cauliflower, eggplant, mushrooms, sauerkraut, spinach, and zucchini, or ½ cup of carrots. Season to taste.

Mixed Salad—An individual-sized salad bowl with three or more of the following: lettuce, tomato (two or three slices), cucumber, celery, radish, carrot, green or

The Prune Pit Seed Story

During the developmental stages of the Big Apple Diet, I accidentally chewed with too much vigor upon a prune that I was eating and ruptured the pit. After evacuating my mouth of the pit debris, a small seed remained, so I ate it. To my surprise, it tasted quite good. So I proceeded to pit and open two more prunes. Again, the seeds were delicious. Every evening for the next two weeks, I would remove the seeds from three prunes and eat them. To my delight, for those two weeks, I lost weight at a more rapid rate than before. I began to suggest the idea to my patients. More than fifty percent of those who ate the prune pit seeds also lost weight more rapidly.

I don't know why it works, but it does. So why not try it—here's how:

After your evening fruit, pit three prunes. Break open the pits with a nutcracker (not your teeth) and eat the seeds. They have a delightful nutty almond taste. Remember, only three prune pit seeds per night, and then only in conjunction with my diet.

I still haven't figured out what to do with the prunes, but one thing is for sure—don't eat 'em.

red pepper, cabbage, scallions, and onion. (Pickles and sauerkraut are permitted, but not recommended because they contain too much salt.) Use dressing described for the lettuce salad at lunch. Toss the salad. It adds bulk and greatly enhances the flavor.

Fruit—One medium-sized orange (recommended), an apple, half of a grapefruit, or half of an average-sized canteloupe. Peel the orange so that the membranes remain intact. Attempt to remove the orange sections without mutilating the fruit. This is fun, it takes time, and more of the fruit's nutrients are retained. Make sure you have your fruit shortly before going to bed. Do not eat it at the midpoint between dinner and retiring as it will tend to start you snacking. A simple rule is to eat the fruit and go to bed. If you retire immediately, you will not eat more food.

Water—Drink from six to eight 8-ounce glasses of liquids daily. Some people require even more. Water is important for the proper functioning of the body, especially the elimination system. Have the water at any time, but make sure you are not using it to appease appetite (see Page 44). In estimating your daily water intake, include **all** beverages, such as coffee, tea, soda, and so forth.

For Goal Weights between 150 and 170 Pounds

Augment dinner by increasing the chicken portion to half of a three- to four-pound chicken.

For Goal Weights over 170 Pounds

Augment dinner by increasing the chicken portion to half of a three- to four-pound chicken. Also, for lunch, substitute one of the following sandwiches for the main luncheon choice:

Egg Sandwich—Hard-boiled (recommended), fried, or scrambled egg, or egg salad with lettuce.

Cheese Sandwich—No more than three slices of cheese (hard only), with lettuce if desired. (See also the last recipe in Chapter Thirteen.)

Tuna Sandwich—Plain tuna with lemon (recommended) or tuna salad, with lettuce if desired.

For the sandwiches, use white, rye, or whole wheat bread, toasted or plain. Avoid "diet" or thin-sliced breads (see the discussion of bread under "Lunch").

And that is it.

Questions and Answers about the Big Apple Diet

Here are some of the questions and answers most often asked about the diet by my beginning diet patients.

Why is chicken such an important part of the diet?

Chicken has many advantages, for the dieter, over other types of protein food:

1. Chicken is a healthful food that contains protein and is relatively low in cholesterol.
2. Chicken can be prepared in a variety of ways.
3. Most people enjoy the taste of chicken.
4. Chicken takes time to eat. Working on the chicken bones will slow you down. Eating slowly not only aids digestion, but it also tends to satisfy.
5. Chicken is easy to digest.
6. Chicken is generally offered at restaurants.
7. Chicken can be cooked and eaten at a later time. One can prepare chicken and use it for from one to three days. This capability makes

chicken especially important to the working homemaker or the single person. It can also be purchased already cooked (barbequed or roasted).

Why chicken only?

I advise that you initially eat only chicken, because after a while you will not think about other foods, and this makes dieting easier. The same helpful principle of sticking to the same diet applies to breakfast and lunch, even though I have included a selection of foods. I find that, as a rule, my most successful patients initially experiment with the breakfast and lunch options, but finally settle down to the same food items day after day. The habit of eating the same food is valuable, for a routine of eating the same meals prevents the imagination from running wild. You are not confronted with limitless culinary choices, thereby conjuring up visions of foods you know you should not eat.

Is eating the same foods daily healthful?

Yes, if you follow my instructions and make sensible choices for breakfast and lunch. Do not choose improper combinations, such as an English muffin for breakfast and a corn muffin for lunch. Even though you will lose weight by doing so, you will be violating the rules of good nutrition. Also, by attempting to placate the appetite by eating "filling foods," you will be defeating your purpose. Remember, appetite is mental, not physical.

Why are there no red meats on your diet?

Generally, I find no fault in red meats—for the nondieter. For the dieter, however, I recommend avoiding them. Red meats are generally higher in calories than chicken, fish, or veal. Red meat seems to be a "starter" food; it seems to stimulate the appetite rather than satisfying it. Many diets recommend four to six ounces of meat for dinner, but this "tease" portion will not satisfy the appetite. On the contrary, it awakens the taste buds and increases the craving for more foods. Have you ever watched a dog being handed a piece of meat or a bone? If so, you are aware that, as the dog eats, it is dangerous to touch him because, even if he is well fed, he acts ravenous and almost frenzied. And he invariably wants more food. Many people react in a similar psychological manner, and if there is anything a dieter does not need, it is increased appetite.

What happens if I get tired of chicken after a week or two?

I find that people who get "tired" of chicken are really tired of making the total effort to lose weight. To test yourself, consider any previous food-oriented diets you have tried. Were you able to stick to any dietary discipline until you lost your excess weight? Probably not. If you will consider the menus offered in Chapter Thirteen, you will realize that there are many and diverse ways of preparing chicken. Getting "bored" is simply an excuse for wanting to cop out. I suggest that you remotivate yourself by reading Chapters Two and Three.

What if I hate chicken?

Start your diet with fish for the first month; then add the veal (or vice versa). It will be a little harder for

you, since fish and veal do not have all the advantages of chicken, but you can still succeed.

How fast can I expect to lose weight on your diet?

The amount and rate of weight loss depends on
many factors, such as the number of pounds by
which one is overweight and daily physical activity.
In general, one can expect a 2 percent to 3 percent
weight loss weekly. Of course, this means that a two-
hundred-pound person will lose more than a one-
hundred-pound one.

The amount of body water plays an important
role in "scale weight." As I point out in greater detail
later, the first week or ten days represents the greatest
weight loss because of water loss. (I recall one very
obese male who lost 25 pounds the first week. This
was simply because he had an unusual amount of
body water. But after several weeks, his weight loss
leveled out to the normal 2 to 3 percent weekly.)

Is it OK to skip breakfast?

No. But not for the reasons you might think. I disagree
strongly with most diet experts, who tell you never to
skip meals because it will make your appetite ravenous by the next meal time and you will end up stuffing yourself. I do not find this to be true, simply because overweight people have big appetites whether
they skip a meal or not. And so what is the advantage of missing a meal? There is none.

But there is a distinct disadvantage. After skipping
a meal, a dieter feels psychologically deprived; there

is a "missing link" in that day's chain of eating. So he subconsciously begins to rationalize that he has earned the right to have another feed before going to bed. The need will overcome him, perhaps after dinner that night, or maybe in the middle of the afternoon **three weeks later.** The reason for this is that we have been conditioned to accept the routine of three meals a day, and, when we miss a meal, the subconsious mind remains aware of the fact—and does not rest until that missing meal is "made up." The problem is that when the missing meal is finally eaten, it not only causes the psychological damage of disrupting the normal eating schedule, but it is liable to contain more calories than the original meal missed.

Remember, most overweight people skip breakfast. Don't be one of them.

How do I handle eating out?

There are times when you will be forced to eat out. Holidays and special occasions make these away-from-home eating experiences inevitable. Summers offer outdoor barbeques. Winters offer family feasts. Even though you have no choice as to the types of foods offered, you **do** have the option as to **quantity.**

Quantity is the key. Take what I call "politely small" portions of the food that the host or hostess has prepared. Common sense and good judgment can resolve what might be a threatening situation if you remember to accent the salads and "lighter" foods.

When it comes to dessert, assuming it is a rich cake or pie, it is not uncommon for dinner guests to smile politely and say, "Just coffee, please." Going to restaurants presents less of a problem. Here your only potential pitfall is looking at a menu, a temptation to be strictly avoided, for the numerous choices described in various styles with different sauces and fillings cause the mouth to water and the imagination to run wild. Remember, **never look at a menu.** Tell the waiter what foods you want. If chicken is not served (in most restaurants, it is on the menu), order broiled fish or veal. Substitute other foods accordingly. Do not use eating out as an excuse to overeat or go off your diet.

What can I do if my appetite flares up and I get hungry?

First, we must define "hunger" and "appetite." Hunger is the body's call for energy. Appetite is the body's call for pleasure. Overweight people have an overabundant supply of body fat that is automatically converted into energy when they are dieting. So, in a sense, overweight people cannot be hungry. What they feel is appetite. As stated before, appetite is the body's call for pleasure. Unfortunately, appetite and hunger are easily confused as they both "feel" the same. So if you "get hungry" when you should not, realize that you are driven by your appetite and ask yourself: "Do I want the immediate pleasure of food or the lifetime pleasure of being thin and more attractive?" When you choose the latter, your "hunger" will magically disappear.

Are diet sodas or low-calorie drinks recommended for quenching thirst?

No, and for good reasons. As hunger is the body's legitimate call for energy, thirst is the legitimate call for water. I learned a startling fact a long time ago: overweight people hate water. Just as they confuse hunger and appetite, they also confuse thirst and appetite. They seek certain liquids as pleasures rather than as necessities. In this sense, overweight people "eat" low-calorie soda and drinks that to them represent instant pleasure and attempt to placate appetite rather than a basic need. They claim that their thirst simply cannot be satisfied by drinking water when the truth is that all one ever really needs to satisfy thirst is water. Nobody ever came crawling off a desert with a parched throat, desperately begging for Diet Pepsi. Another reason not to drink diet soft drinks is that they, especially colas, contain salt, and salt retains water. I believe that if every overweight person were to stop drinking diet sodas, the companies would go out of business. Think about it. How many thin people do you know who drink diet soft drinks?

CHAPTER SIX
Directing Your Mind

Up to this point I have discussed the physical and psychological aspects of eating and dieting. Now you are going to learn how to direct your mind and to apply the concepts you have learned in previous chapters. The tool you need is Hypnosis II, a do- it-yourself method of self-suggestion, which is really a way to train yourself to behave the way you want to behave. It is different from traditional hypnosis or self-hypnosis, as you will learn. In addition to helping you with weight control, it can be a useful tool for helping you get many of the things you want out of life. It is **not** a trick or a gimmick, it is a genuinely effective technique that you can master readily and use successfully with great pleasure.

How I Developed Hypnosis II

I had considerable training and experience as a hypnotist when I was young, but there had been no occasion to use it when I went into professional practice. One day I happened to pick up a book on the subject, and it occurred to me that this might be a great way to help patients lose weight.

Much to my surprise, I experienced little success in hypnotizing patients. After a session, many complained of not "feeling" hypnotized. Upon returning for their next session, others would tell me that they had actually eaten more than before. What was wrong with hypnosis? After a good deal of thought, I finally concluded that previous hypnotic subjects were not defending prior subconscious habits, such as overeating. They were simply being hypnotized for the fun of it. So they "let go" and were easily hypnotized.

Consider the same hypnotizable subject as a patient in a professional office. Although the conscious mind is willing, the subconscious mind is on guard. It wants to retain eating habits and views hypnosis and the hypnotist as a threat to its (the subconscious') existence. This defensive attitude prevents most people from being hypnotized. Or they resist out of fear that another person would control their minds.

I investigated regular self-hypnosis that did not work, either, and for the same reasons. My frustration led me to develop a different version, which I call

Hypnosis II. From the very first, it worked wonders. Hypnosis II is simple, and it can be readily learned without professional help. This chapter offers all necessary instructions.

Learning about Hypnosis II

Hypnosis II is a self-induced state of profound relaxation, in which the subconscious mind will accept suggestions a thousand times more readily than during ordinary states of awareness. Relaxation is a normal and natural mental state in which one is more open to suggestion. Salesmen instinctively know, for example, that, if they can make their customers relax through dining or entertainment, they stand a better chance of selling their products. This same type of relaxation may occur when watching a movie. People get so emotionally involved with the drama that they actually weep. Hypnosis II is simply a way to control this natural emotional susceptibility, and allow us to receive specific suggestions that accord with our own desires. It differs from hypnosis or self-hypnosis in that there is no trance or need to concentrate.

A state of trance or deep concentration alerts the subconscious, makes it defensive, and blocks suggestion. Hypnosis II "catches" the subconscious off guard, and so suggestion can be implanted easily.

Before getting into Hypnosis II techniques, it might be well to step back for a moment and discuss some basics that will help you to use Hypnosis II with maximum effectiveness.

Understanding Suggestion

From birth on, people are constantly subjected to suggestions. They are taught formally and informally by family, friends, and society. A television food commercial, for example, can make your mouth water. Most of all, people are subjected to suggestion by themselves—by their own misapprehensions, fears, insecurities, and desires.

Levels of Mental Functions

Most people are aware, of course, that the mind functions on two levels, the conscious and the subconscious. The conscious mind deals with our overt desires, observations, and feelings. It is the surface mind, the voluntary mind. People who look into a mirror and say, "I'd give anything to have a slim, attractive body, to lose this ugly excess flesh," are governed by the surface mind.

The conscious mind also governs imagination and rationality. Human beings are the only creatures on earth possessing the unique ability, consciously, to be aware, think, reason, connect ideas, form judgments, and the like.

The Subconscious Mind

If the conscious mind is the tip of the mental iceberg, the subconscious is the huge, unexposed portion beneath the water. The subconscious is the hidden mind that often controls us without our knowledge.

Buried in its depths are our unacknowledged thoughts, ideas, and beliefs. Among its other functions, the subconscious governs the learning we acquire through repetition. The routines we follow and the automatic responses we make are learned information stored in the subconscious mind. Advertising people use repetition to achieve recognition. Commercials are repeated many times until we subconsciously get the message. We automatically absorb hundreds of ideas or suggestions without realizing what has happened.

A healthy mind reflects a balance between the conscious and the subconscious. All too often, however, the two are in conflict. We are pulled in one direction by our conscious mind and in another by the subconscious.

The greater the conflict, the greater the likelihood of mental or emotional upset. The subconscious mind of someone who has been smoking for twenty to thirty years, for example, totally accepts the fact that smoking is pleasurable. Warned against smoking by doctors and government reports, the smoker accepts that advice consciously. Efforts to stop smoking, however, are completely unsuccessful. The larger and more powerful subconscious mind overrides the conscious decision to stop smoking, however unhealthy the effects. The subconscious desire to smoke is too strong. This explains why so many smokers continue to smoke, even when they feel disgusted and say they want to stop. The key to overcoming any bad habit—and the specific purpose of Hypnosis II—is to retrain the subconscious mind.

The information you have gleaned so far about overweight has dealt mainly with voluntary or conscious control. Although we have little contact with our subconscious minds (occasionally we do, via dreams or inspiration), we know that the subconscious reinforces our pleasure in eating and that we will have to confront these subconscious feelings in order to change them.

Take the example of Fred that follows. It shows both the different ways the conscious and the subconscious work and the need to deal with a weight problem on both levels before one can hope to achieve a desired goal.

Fred claimed that, "I've been trying to lose weight all my life. I've seen every 'fat doctor' I could find. None of them has helped me. So I'm going to try one more time. You're my last resort." (My thought at this point was that it is interesting to note how people never blame themselves for their plight.)

In machine-gun fashion, he continued, "The reason I can't stick to any diet is because whenever I start I get terrible headaches. In addition to those doctors, I've seen neurologists, endocrinologists, and even spent three months on a psychiatrist's couch trying to get rid of these diet headaches. But nobody could help me."

Fred began to talk more softly and quietly. "I have a responsible position and work with numbers all day—columns and columns and pages and pages of tiny, but very important, figures. My work is exacting and full of tension. I really do want to lose weight, but I simply cannot function with headaches. On your diet, doctor, can you guarantee that I won't get them?"

Let us pause for a moment and analyze Fred's problem. First, there were his vital statistics. He stood five feet ten inches tall, was almost forty years old (he looked fifty), and used the complete capacity of my office scale, which was 360 pounds (163.6 kilos). His attitude was extremely defensive. From his history, I knew that both of his parents had been fat and that he had been overweight all of his childhood and adult life. He admitted that he loved food and loved to eat. It was obvious to me that Fred's subconscious love of food was even stronger than his conscious desire to lose weight. Every time he attempted a diet, his subconscious mind did everything it could to defeat him. The tool that Fred's subconscious used was, of course, headaches, a perfect weapon, for how could a person who works with "tiny" figures and tension hope to function with headaches? Fred subconsciously created headaches in order to justify his diet failures.

This explanation probably seems elementary and obvious. But for Fred it was extremely difficult to accept. I told him that in my view he was at a major crossroad in his life and that, if he wanted to succeed, he would have to do exactly what I told him. Fred agreed, but shook his head skeptically when I outlined what I expected of him. I told him that on my program he would probably have headaches for about a week or two, but with Hypnosis II and a clear, conscious understanding of what he was doing, we would probably be able to lick the problem.

Fred stuck to our arrangement and successfully lost weight; the headaches lasted only three days.

Hypnosis II

Now it is time to take a closer look at Hypnosis II. There are two basic steps, neither of which has any value without the other:

1. Induction—a. The act of producing a relaxed state.
              b. The technique of increasing it
2. Programming—Giving the necessary suggestions.

When asked how Hypnosis II induction feels, people answer in different words. But, without exception, their descriptions are all positive; I have never heard a patient describe the experience as negative or frightening. The most common descriptions are wonderful, restful, peaceful, serene. In addition to this feeling of euphoria, three sensations are generally experienced: relaxation, heaviness, and indifference.

To experience all three feelings would be ideal, but any one or any combination will suffice. The objective in experiencing these mental states is to let the individual gain access to the subconscious mind.

Induction—Step 1a

The process is simple and peaceful. No strain, effort, or tension is involved. Be seated in a not-too-comfortable chair, for that might induce sleep. Lying down is not recommended for the same reason. Do not seek a quiet place, for the sounds of life around you will play an important role in your Hypnosis II induction. The only thing you must insist upon is privacy.

Place your unclenched hands and lower arms on your thighs and close your eyes. Relax. Don't try to feel the effect. Many beginners try to produce a special feeling; they don't know what it is, but they try for it anyway. Don't. You don't even have to concentrate. In simple fact, the exact reverse is true: the more you try to concentrate, the more you tense your mind and the more difficult it becomes to reach the subconscious mind.

Just sit and let your mind wander. That's right—**wander.** Think about anything that comes into your mind. Even if negative thoughts enter your consciousness, that won't hinder you. As you sit there, eyes closed, with your hands in your lap, become aware of the sounds both inside and outside of the room. It's truly amazing how acute our auditory sense becomes when our eyes are closed. Perhaps you'll hear the sound of a ticking clock. Or perhaps car engines and horns. Or people conversing, children laughing, dogs barking.

Pick a sound, or several sounds, and listen to them. After two to three minutes you'll find that your body will start to relax, to feel loose and limp. Continue to listen to these sounds and focus part of your attention on your legs. Remember, do not concentrate. By simply thinking of your legs, you'll begin to feel them becoming more and more relaxed. The sensation will be similar to the feeling you get after taking a long walk and then sitting down. By thinking of your legs as "tired," they become the simplest part of your anatomy to relax. Once you have achieved what you considered to be optimum leg relaxation, mentally label this state **Alpha**.

Alpha is a code word which in your future Hypnosis II sessions will always be associated with leg relaxation. After you become proficient at Hypnosis II, all you'll have to do is think of the code word Alpha and your legs will relax. We call this **immediate induction**.

Now, focus upon your arms. As you did with your legs, begin to imagine your arms becoming very relaxed. Once this happens, label the relaxed state with the code word **Beta**.

Next, relax your head and face by thinking about your scalp, brow, and eyelids. Unclench your teeth and swallow. For mouth relaxation, use the code word **Gamma**.

Your final focus will be on your torso. Begin with the back of your neck and shoulders, and proceed with the rest of your body. Use the code word **Delta** once torso relaxation is accomplished.

Don't have any fear that the code words Alpha, Beta, Gamma, or Delta can have any strange or magical effect simply by being spoken; they will take effect only when you are performing Hypnosis II, and at no other time.

Patients always ask me how much time they will have to devote to this first part of the Induction process. Initially, the time varies with the individual. One may spend anywhere from five to ten minutes when starting to practice Hypnosis II. But once the proper mind set has been established, it can be done as fast as one can say Alpha, Beta, Gamma, Delta.

Induction—Step 1b

The next part in induction is to deepen the state by creating a feeling of heaviness. This is an easy state to attain, for it is a direct result of relaxation. In other words, once you become relaxed, your body will automatically become "comfortably heavy." However, to aid the process, we use **fantasy.**

In Hypnosis II, fantasy redirects the mind from its natural state of awareness and the flow of conscious thought. The one firm rule is that the fantasy should be pleasant and embrace happy thoughts. Any subject upon which you can fantasize with pleasure is legitimate. The best fantasies come from your own mind, but if you are at a loss as to where to begin, try the one described next, modifying it as it suits your fancy. Remember, do not concentrate or try too hard. Relax. Let your mind flow instead of trying to control its direction.

A Fantasy (Example)

Begin by seeing yourself, actually feeling your body, in a comfortable rocking chair. You're on a beautiful park lawn. The temperature is very comfortable, about 75 degrees, and it's a beautiful spring or summer day. You're rocking s-l-o-w-l-y back and forth. As you glance upward, you see that the sky is a magnificent blue, with small puffs of clouds that remind you of cotton balls. You are very happy. You become aware of the aroma of freshly cut grass. (Many patients who have tried this fantasy tell me that they can actually smell the grass.)

As you look down, you see that the lawn has just been mowed. You continue rocking, and this rocking motion relaxes you even more. You hear the pleasant sound of leaves rustling in a gentle breeze; you look up and see the heavy foliage. Now you look at the grass again and see that the sun shining through the leaves is creating magnificent shadow art. You are enjoying this blissful feeling more and more as you continue to rock, s-l-o-w-l-y, back and forth, s-l-o-w-l-y back and forth, and now you close your eyes and become totally relaxed, with a sensation of bodily heaviness.

You have now reached the third sensation in induction—that of becoming indifferent. You aren't sleeping. You're totally aware of your surroundings. Mentally you're quite alert; yet you don't care. Now you have achieved a perfect Hypnosis II induction, and are ready for programming.

Programming—Step 2

Programming is the second half of Hypnosis II. It is the act of giving yourself proper suggestions for weight loss. The way to successful programming is the formulation and phrasing of realistic and workable suggestions. Here are examples of **incorrect** suggestions that should be avoided.

1. **I dislike fattening foods.** There is no way that an overweight person who enjoys eating will ever dislike fattening foods.

2. **I love nonfattening foods.** Again, this is impossible. I have yet to find an overweight person who can be satisfied or feel "filled up" on a bowl of sauerkraut or lettuce. Even the much touted "diet malted," which consists of skim milk, saccharin, chopped ice, and vanilla extract tastes like a barium (chalk) cocktail after a while.

3. **I will stick to my diet.** Overweight people will stick to a diet only if the proper motivation is provided. To suggest that they will stick to a diet on any other basis is like planting a flower seed in wet cement and expecting it to grow.

Here are some **correct** suggestions. When you have read them, compare them to the incorrect ones, and see the difference.

1. **I desire to be more attractive than I am presently.**

2. **Since being more attractive means being slim, I want to be slim.**

3. **Since being slim means eating less food, I will stick to my diet.**

Once the Hypnosis II programming is set, it, too, can be summarized in a single word, a word that summarizes the three proper diet suggestions. If that seems improbable, consider for a moment the word "lion." Your mind produces numerous images: a large, catlike beast, with a mane, roaming the jungles; the king of beasts, a killer, dangerous, possessing a mighty roar. All of these ideas are included in the mental images your mind automatically and randomly conjures up in a split second in response to the word lion.

This same principle of immediate association is used in Hypnosis II. The word I use is **Omega**. Just as the word lion produces a number of visual images and emotions, so will Omega trigger the diet suggestions as well as the ideas presented in this book—the mental texture or flavor of the concepts you have learned.

To help this process, it is a good idea to memorize the diet suggestions, which serve as a reminder of all you have learned and which Omega will bring promptly to mind. Here they are again:

1. I desire to be more attractive than I am presently.

2. Since being attractive means being slim, I want to be slim.

3. Since being slim means eating less food, I will stick to my diet.

In summary, the word Omega as used with Hypnosis II means:

MORE ATTRACTIVE——THIN——PROPER DIET

The Hypnosis II technique is simple. Relax with the code words Alpha, Beta, Gamma, and Delta, which combine with the fantasy to create body heaviness. Program yourself with the word Omega. It should be spoken silently, not aloud. Repeat Omega seven times. (Seven is generally the number of repetitions required to impress the subconscious mind deeply.)

Ending your Hypnosis II Session

To end Hypnosis II, count one... two... three... very slowly, then open your eyes. You will be back in your natural state of awareness. You'll feel rested and relaxed. There will be no emotional or physical price to pay. You will have succeeded in planting constructive suggestions in your subconscious so that it will now work to help you.

Questions and Answers about Hypnosis II

I am invariably asked four questions about Hypnosis II:

How often should I practice Hypnosis II?

You should hold two sessions every day—upon awakening and before retiring and at **no other time.** The first session will help relax you during your waking hours, and the second session will promote a good night's sleep.

Do not practice Hypnosis II more than twice daily. If you do, you will exhaust the subconscious mind, and it will rebel by blocking the suggestions. The mind will no longer "hear" them. Many diet clubs tell members to paste an unflattering photograph of themselves on the refrigerator door as a reminder of why they should not open it if they are tempted to make unauthorized visits to the refrigerator. The gimmick, and that is all it is, works for a day or two, but after a while the photograph "disappears" as the subconscious mind blocks it out. So do not abuse Hypnosis II by overuse.

Should I continue Hypnosis II after I attain my goal weight?

Yes I suggest practicing for the remainder of your life. Daily sessions reinforce the subconscious mind to remain thin. Since it is simple to perform and requires little time, why stop?

There is an additional benefit in Hypnosis II. The morning session relaxes body and mind, producing a restful state which prepares you for the day's activities. The evening session tends to invite a restful night's sleep. Personally, I have used Hypnosis II for the past 18 years and have easily kept off the one hundred pounds that I originally lost.

Do I have to "believe" in or have "faith" in Hypnosis II to make it work?

No. Hypnosis II is not a cult practiced by fanatics. It's based on sound theory and solid experience repeated over many years. We live successfully (and sometimes unsuccessfully) because of suggestions that affect our everyday actions and thoughts. From the first rap on the behind at birth, we are bombarded with suggestions. We are conditioned by our parents, our teachers, our society, or religious leaders, and our peers. We **learn** our concepts. We are not born with them. And Hypnosis II is simply a method of accepting suggestion by practice and thus **learning**, as opposed to faith or belief.

Can I follow the Big Apple Diet without using Hypnosis II?

Yes. Even without Hypnosis II, the Big Apple Diet is still the easiest reducing diet there is.

Can I use Hypnosis II for other problems?

Of course. And remember, you will be on your own, as this book deals only with controlling overweight. Since Hypnosis II is harmless, however, you can experiment to your heart's content. The main point to remember is to use suggestions that are realistic and workable.

A word of caution: Do not combine losing weight with another problem, such as quitting cigarette smoking. Such an effort will only lessen the total effect.

A Final Word

To ensure success, be patient. Do not try too hard, or look for immediate change in your attitude toward eating. Remember, your "overeating mind" has probably been functioning for many years. Give it time to change, **and change it will.**

CHAPTER SEVEN
Twelve Positive Pointers

On Formal Exercise

Most reducing programs tell you to exercise on a regular basis and "tighten up those loose muscles." Physical exertion is supposed to help you lose weight, look thinner and feel better. But this is an oversimplification, and often a great mistake. Formal exercise, like jogging or calisthenics, may be wrong for the dieter because regular exercise is simply another problem and another feeling of failure. I have seen it happen hundreds of times. The exercise cult has cost these people money and misery, and it has not helped their basic problem at all.

Frequently dieters enroll in a formal exercise program and do well for the first week or ten days, carried on the wings of inspiration and hope. Then they abruptly stop. They simply cannot keep it up because they do not enjoy it. The answer is that simple. It is no fun at all. I have learned that such people simply will not exercise on a regular basis. Those who try to do so, out of a sense of guilt or desperation, only add to their unhappiness an additional burden of guilt for failing to "keep up the good work."

This, in turn, brings in its wake a level of dejection or depression that can only be soothed by heavy eating. For the very few who stick to a formal exercise program, there exists another psychological pitfall: They feel a slight hardening of the body, begin to think they are thin, and let down their guard. They fall into the same trap of eating more than they should.

I once worked with a 200-pound woman whose goal weight was 120. She was doing very well and had lost 50 pounds. All of a sudden, her progress stopped. I was puzzled. There was no apparent reason. Then I learned that, when she had lost 50 pounds, her father had given her an exercise machine, which she began to use. The combination of having to do two things that she really disliked (eating less **and** exercising) proved too much for her. Dieting was difficult enough. I convinced her to get rid of the exercise machine, and she went right back to losing weight.

Physical activity is splendid, and exercise is extremely important to one's health. But formal exercise is not the answer for people who are overweight.

With regard to formal exercise, be aware that some health spas, figure salons, and health clubs push for yearly contracts with payment in advance, knowing that most of the people who join will not fulfill their contracts. As a matter of simple fact, if all **did** remain for the year, the club would need a physical plant the size of the Roman Coliseum. Anyone who has visited an exercise club for more than a week will surely have noticed a small group of regulars. These are the hard-core exercise buffs who enjoy body building and formal working out.

The average overweight person is not interested, and the exercise can be psychologically detrimental. Heavy physical expenditure of energy causes a great loss of water (greater for those with excess weight). After working out at the gym, such people may jump on the scale and discover a weight loss of four or five pounds. They reward themselves by going out to eat. When their tissues return to normal (that is, when they have regained water loss) they are back where they started or possibly a step backward from renewed overeating. If you want to try a gym, find one that will allow you to pay by the week, or at most by the month.

What should dieters do for exercise? In my case, when I set out to lose weight I enjoyed walking (window-shopping is great), playing tennis, and bicycle riding. I did no one activity to the point of exhaustion, but used each for social pleasure as well as exercise.

On Fasting

Many diet specialists offer fasts, that is, "starvation diets" of less than two hundred calories a day, as a method of losing weight. Essentially the diet consists of fruit juices and liquids. Such diets do result in loss of weight, often quick loss, but they do not keep weight off. The minute the fat person leaves the controlled environment of the fast, the weight is regained.

In my opinion, fasting is a gimmick and definitely not an eating pattern with the psychological assurance of a purposeful routine. The accent is on how rapidly the weight loss occurs, whereas the real question should be, "How do I keep off the weight I lose?"

Many find fasting appealing. They are excited by the prospect of large weight losses and think it is easier to stop eating altogether than to control what they eat. But fast weight loss is at best a temporary measure. Let me give you an example.

A young couple, married for two years, came to me for help. The husband was 125, and the wife about 100, pounds overweight. They'd met at a well-known medical clinic, where each had come to take off weight on a diet fast in which they ate no solid food. They met toward the end of their fasts, when they had taken off considerable weight and were at their most attractive. They fell in love and were married. Within a year after they had left the confines of the clinic, they had regained the lost weight. When they came to my office, they were both unhappy, not only with themselves but with each other. I explained that they had met at the equivalent of a masquerade party and that their real identities had gradually become exposed after they were married. I pointed out that each had looked to the other as an ideal: a thin person. Now they had to accept each other as each actually was, and neither one liked it. They would both have to work at becoming thin—not in a sudden dramatic fast, but on a properly self-motivated diet by which they would gradually take off weight and keep it off. Currently, they are progressing beautifully, and a happy ending seems to be in sight.

On the "Ten-Pound Syndrome"

The "ten-pound syndrome" is a common experience. All dieters take off approximately ten pounds quite quickly after which their rate of weight loss slows down sharply. That ten pounds should be such a common denominator seems strange. To a person who is twenty pounds overweight, it represents 50 percent of the desired weight loss. To a person who is a hundred pounds overweight, it represents only 10 percent of the desired weight loss. It does not matter. "Ten pounds" has a kind of magic. People become excited, inspired by this evidence of progress. Feeling more attractive, they let down their guard. The result is that they begin to overeat again.

An understanding of why it is so easy to lose the first ten pounds will help you avoid this common trap.

When we start to diet, the result of the first week's effort is usually a loss of five to ten pounds. Unfortunately, this loss is about 80 percent water rather than fatty tissue. The person who does not know this is likely to become cocky, expecting to lose a similar amount every week. This simply will not happen, and knowing that fact will keep you from building up false hopes.

Women retain water just prior to and during menstruation. Many women use this fact as an excuse to eat, however, since they are "going to gain weight anyway." If you stick to your eating plan, you will lose the weight both in water and fatty tissue at the termination of the menstrual cycle.

An interesting aspect of the ten-pound syndrome is that almost 50 percent of the people I have worked with, after losing the first ten pounds, say of themselves in complete seriousness, "When I was fat." On many, the weight loss is scarcely discernible. One way to avoid this common error is to keep a firm goal in mind. If, for example, you eventually plan to weigh 175 pounds, make up your mind that you can say "when I was fat" **only** when you weigh 175 pounds.

On Gimmicks

Some diet organizations advise you to put pictures of yourself on the refrigerator or notes on the bathroom mirror to remind yourself that you are fat. Another suggestion is that you write down the precise weight you want to be and paste it at various visible points around the house. This may sound like a good idea, but it is not. Actually, it is a complete waste of time. One soon learns to ignore such notes and treat them as if they do not even exist. The human mind simply has a way of not seeing things it does not want to see. The best way to help yourself stay on your diet is sincere motivation.

On Chewing Gum

There is a commonly accepted myth that chewing gum decreases the appetite. This is not true. The habit of chewing gum is a potential bomb since chewing tends to reinforce the oral habit by keeping the mouth active and increasing salivation. Ideally, people will learn to control oral habits as they follow a diet. Chewing gum is to eaters what plastic cigarettes are to would-be nonsmokers. They do not help.

On the Unit Theory

It's important for overweight people to understand that they eat in units. If there is a quart of ice cream around, somehow one does not feel satisfied until the whole quart is gone. The solution is to use the unit factor in a positive way. One egg is one unit. To fry that egg means you will eat just that one egg. But serving several scrambled eggs is a completely different matter; there is no way to judge the unit of a single egg, and so one tends to eat more.

The same principle applies to dry cereal. The odds are great that if a person measures an ounce from a large box of cereal, he or she will take more as a second serving. The solution? Buy individual servings, which contain approximately one ounce. Cheese, to give another example, should never be bought in slabs or chunks but already sliced. In other words, buy as many foods already packaged in individual units or servings as possible. Or, for economy's sake, the dieter can create a supply of individual servings ahead of time by dividing large chunks or units (such as slabs of cheese).

On Compensating for Overeating

Eat on a regular schedule as often as possible. If you are forced, through travel or vacation or some social event, to eat more during a certain day or period, do not try to compensate. Never try to make up the day after for the steak dinner with all the trimmings that you ate the evening before. If you stuff at lunch, do not try to punish yourself by eating less at dinner. This practice never seems to work out. Simply eat the same amount at supper as if you had had your regular lunch. This will avoid feelings of guilt and let you maintain the important psychological confidence that comes from regularity in your eating habits.

On Eating with "Normal People"

When eating with a nondieting friend, it is not necessary to explain your order. Experience has taught me that even friends react strangely to people on diets. They try to persuade you to order everything on the menu, tell you that you are looking thin and can afford a binge, and come up with numerous other arguments aimed at getting you to stuff yourself on the fattening special of the day. The best explanation about your not eating much is no explanation at all. Usually you will not be questioned unless you make a fuss about what you are eating. But, if you are questioned, simply say you are not hungry.

On the Coffee Break

The coffee break may appear to be no more than a ten-minute snack somewhere between breakfast and lunch. Actually, it is a barometer of one's attitude toward food and a daily testing time. It requires great restraint for any office worker not to join the large group that eagerly descends to the company cafeteria or greets the mobile "coffee cart" laden with goodies. Exercising such self-control is even harder for people who especially enjoy eating.

The coffee break is neither fish nor fowl; it means different things to different people. To the thin, busy executive it may mean a cup of black coffee, drunk at the desk. To another person it means something else entirely. It means coffee AND. The AND can be anything: a danish, cookies, cake, even a sandwich. Since the overweight person associates "coffee" with coffee and solid foods, attempting to drink coffee by itself triggers the appetite for something to eat with it. This is why I recommend avoiding coffee, or any other beverage except water, between meals. There are, however, social situations which make it almost necessary to eat or drink. If you are invited to a friend's house for "coffee," you will almost surely be served cake or cookies as well.

Refusing everything would make you stand out like a sore thumb and make it obvious that you were on a diet, leading to a "diet discussion"—something to be avoided. So it is perfectly permissible to have a single cup of coffee or other beverage as described in Chapter Five. Realizing that you are not placating appetite but simply conforming to social amenities will let you enjoy the coffee without any feeling of guilt.

Guarded Enthusiasm

Optimism should be the dieter's natural outlook, but do not make the mistake of red-hot exuberance and dash into your diet like an undisciplined racehorse. Fanatical enthusiasm burns itself out. It resembles starting a mile race by sprinting at top speed, guaranteeing that you will run down before you reach your goal. My heart sinks when I meet an about-to-diet person who is out of control with excitement, who vows to follow every requirement of the diet with religious fervor. I have learned that such fanatics always wilt quickly. Within two weeks their emotions have burned out, and they no longer follow their diets.

On Giving in to Temptation

When overcome by temptation, one should give in and consciously break the diet regimen. Or, simply, eat and enjoy it. This is far superior to surrendering, after fighting it off, to a long suppressed urge for cake or pie or whatever and then feeling terribly guilty afterward. Guilt leads to depression, and depression to a sense of futility. It is better to enjoy the indiscretion. Of course, you must realize that you cannot indulge yourself this way all the time. The ideal is perfect self-control. But, if you do slip once in a while, remember you are only human and may be allowed an occasional mistake.

I recently averaged the weight of a group of thin people who visited my office for reasons other than losing weight. I discovered that their weekly weight fluctuated an average of three pounds. This obviously means that thin people overeat occasionally, but they have the ability to return to proper eating patterns. Others must develop this same ability.

Guarded enthusiasm is economical use of emotion. It is easy to maintain, just as it is easier to trot than to sprint. You can travel much farther that way, and it fosters patience and persistence in achieving your goal.

On Being Silent

I recently attended a wedding. A psychologist and his wife sat at my table. She was on a diet and let everybody know it from the moment we sat down. Not only did she bore everyone at the table, including her husband, with her "fat" talk, but she constantly offered food she would not eat to the other guests. "Does anyone want my potatoes? Here, have my bread, my dessert." The woman did not realize that her actions were detrimental to her diet.

Do not talk about your diet. Keep it private. First of all, "diet" is a word that simply does not get the proper respect from many thin people. They consider heart trouble and diabetes serious matters and will caution you not to eat foods that might aggravate your illness. But obesity is not taken seriously. Secondly, talking about what you intend to do dissipates, or wastes, your energy. If you keep talking about doing something, you will suddenly find that you have "talked it out." You no longer have the drive to act. If, on the other hand, you keep your goal to yourself, it will be like a concentrated mental vitamin that constantly imparts energy to motivate you.

A third reason for silence is that constant talk about your good intentions will lead you, unconsciously, to make your diet look larger and more difficult than it really is, and you will become discouraged as a result. A fourth reason is that people you know may interfere with your progress, either by doubting your ability or poking fun at you. A further reason is that people tend to play amateur psychologist. They'll "analyze" your motives—your problems, your strong and weak points, your deep inner reasons for wanting to lose weight—and in the process, they may confuse you as to your goal, which is to substitute the pleasure of being thin and attractive for the pleasure of eating.

If you feel like talking about being on a diet, ask yourself this question. Is it possible that I am not really serious, that I want to be discouraged, that I am perhaps looking for someone to blame for making me lose heart, rather than facing my own lack of determination? A final and practical reason for silence is that, if you do not live up to your stated ambition, you will not look foolish.

CHAPTER EIGHT
Games Dieters Play

Some dieters are made of firm stuff. They hold rigorously to necessary dietary procedures and make tangible gains with no delay. Sadly, such "ideal" dieters comprise only a small percentage of those who attempt to follow weight-loss programs. The others run into difficulty. It is tough to pass up that large piece of chocolate cake, that Sunday morning habit of sausages and pancakes, that before-going-to-bed habit of something sweet and fattening washed down with a big glass of milk. It is a battle. But that battle can be won. I have seen thousands of patients who successfully fought their way through the temptations of habit and of "friends" offering them gifts of fattening foods and through the appetite pangs that seem to have an imagination of their own—an imagination that conjures up images of whatever you like best to eat.

Once in a while, we slip. As we climb toward our goal, we slip to one knee and grab a quick candy bar or go on a binge of eating the fattening foods that haunt our dreams. As we have said, one can give in to temptation once in a while. This chapter is not concerned with the weak moments we all seem to experience. It deals with deliberate subterfuges and mental games that dieters play to avoid facing their own responsibility.

The games have one thing in common. They all involve lying to yourself. That is pretty hard language, but softer words are no favor to you. These are the games you must stop playing before you can diet successfully. If you come across one you have tried, recognize it and avoid it from here on. You will be better equipped to get back on the right track and on with your diet.

Searching for a Miracle

This is a way to avoid serious and disciplined dieting by literally trying everything—every new book, every fad. The purpose, ostensibly, is to find a combination of foods that will satisfy appetite and help lose weight. Unfortunately, this miracle diet does not exist because no diet by itself will appease appetite. Only a diet combined with proper motivation will work. So the miracle seeker rarely pursues any one diet for longer than a week or two. This is a garden-variety case of self-deception, following the carrot on a stick that you know you will never reach.

The Cure: Simply realize that you are kidding yourself, that leaping from diet A to B and then to diets Y and Z is exactly the same as not-dieting at all. You are avoiding the fact that a diet without proper motivation is a waste of time. I suggest looking in the mirror and saying to yourself in a firm voice, "I will stop looking for miracles, and get down to business."

"All or Nothing"

This game is played with, say, a box of cookies. Tom, a cookie fiend, eats one chocolate chip cookie, then another, and another. When he has devoured about half the contents of the box, he tells himself he might as well finish the whole thing and get rid of it. Then he will not be tempted later.

The Cure: Realize that the cookie box will never be empty because there is always another box— today, tomorrow, and forever. If Tom had really wanted to "get rid of" the cookies, he could have thrown them out.

Shopping for Someone Else

This is a favorite game of supermarket shoppers. They fill their baskets with fattening foods, telling them-selves that they are buying these goodies for some-one else. The forthcoming visit of a friend or relative is always a good excuse. Or, one can always cook up the excuse that it is for one's husband or wife, who has been working so hard. Guess who ends up eating the shopping bag full of chocolate chip cookies, candy bars, ice cream, and assorted tidbits?

The Cure: If Uncle Harry or Aunt Harriet really are coming for a visit, base your shopping on exactly the amount of time they will be staying and the exact number of meals you will be preparing. Then write out a specific shopping list and follow it to the letter in the supermarket. Incidentally, most people like chicken. So you will be able to serve it in several ways to your visitor. And whatever you cook for such guests, should they not like chicken, you can always have a chicken already cooked for yourself, so that you will not be forced to vary your diet so much.

Gorging

You have a powerful appetite, say, for seven-layer cake. This is your private dream, your secret lust. So far you have denied yourself, but your mind has not stopped working on the problem. Success! One day you discover a marvelous way to eat all of the seven-layer cake you want; in fact, the more you eat the better. You are "punishing" yourself by stuffing your stomach so full of the stuff that you will become physically ill. Playing such a dirty trick on yourself will cure you of ever wanting to touch the stuff again. You go ahead and eat without guilt, and, to your joy, you are "cured." You do not want any more seven-layer cake—at least not for the next twenty-four hours. Then the urge returns as strongly as ever!

The Cure: If a vision of any food is driving you crazy, you have a simple choice: either fight and win a battle to overcome the temptation, or succumb in a common sense way by allowing yourself an exception, a moment of weakness, and having a portion of the "forbidden fruit." Then make a fresh start by getting right back into the regimen of your regular diet.

Show Business

This man or woman is playing a dramatic game and using the world as a captive audience. He wears a long, mournful expression before family and friends. He eats "like a bird," ordering small portions and picking at them, usually leaving part of the food untouched on his plate. He does not seem to lose weight, however, and, as a result, is a topic of conversation and sympathy. "Poor George. He eats like a bird, but his triple chin and huge belly just won't shrink. It must be an unfortunate case of metabolism." Poor George is not to be pitied. He is as fat as ever because he is playing the hypocrite by starving himself in front of any audience and stuffing himself in private.

Or, take the case of Betty. Betty was a happily married, thirty-five-year-old mother of two. She "dramatized" herself into becoming thirty pounds overweight. As a member of a weekly group therapy session on weight control, she insisted that she never ate much and simply could not understand why she remained fat. The other members of the group were completely sympathetic, for whenever they all dined together Betty hardly ate.

One day I visited Betty when she was ill. She needed a towel and asked me to take one from a dresser drawer. Not only did I find the towel, but I also found two boxes of pretzels and potato chips carefully tucked away.

George and Betty sneak food. They stuff themselves with cakes, cookies, and candy, but cannot
bring themselves to admit it. I am convinced that
many people like George and Betty are really convinced that they do not sneak extra food. To accuse
them directly is to wound their sensibilities and rouse
wide-eyed protestations of innocence and accusa-
tions that you are being unjust.

The Cure: Admitting self-deceit can be difficult. But
once you admit it, be kind. Do not berate yourself or
feel disgusted. Remember that you **can** change.

Special Occasions

Maude sticks to her diet religiously until a "special
occasion" comes up at which it is socially proper and
necessary to "eat with the group" at a party or in a
restaurant. On such occasions she eats anything she
wants and as much of it as she can hold. What is the
problem? With her attitude, the special occasions
grow and grow—from holidays and birthdays to a
"lunch" with a girl in the office Maude barely knows
to celebrate her engagement to a man Maude will
never meet. Maude soon becomes more social than
ever, joining groups and making many new friends.
Such social activity is a thin subterfuge for finding
more "special occasions" as excuses to eat heartily
and without restraint.

The Cure: Take a simple hard look at yourself
and what you are doing. How many of the new
"friends" do you really like or have anything in common with? If no food were involved, would you really

consider them interesting? Stop before you go on eating binges to celebrate such "special occasions" as your cat's birthday.

Exercising It off

This is a useful bit of nonsense to hand oneself while sneaking guiltily home from the supermarket with a bag loaded with the wrong foods. Then, as you bite into that second slab of apple pie topped with ice cream, you tell yourself it is perfectly all right. You vow silently (you cannot speak aloud because your cheeks are stuffed with pie), "I'll begin exercising tomorrow." Spurred by guilt, city dwellers envision jogging through the city streets; homeowners imagine doing calisthenics or performing distasteful physical chores around the house, such as that long-delayed obligation to clean out the garage. All such guilt-fed determination dies by the light of dawn.

The Cure: If you hate exercise, face the fact. It is that simple. Ask yourself if you have ever kept a desperate promise to exercise in the past. If not, why believe that you will change your basic way of life tomorrow?

Exercise is best used for body conditioning, in any case, and not for weight loss. To lose just one pound, you must expend 3,500–4000 calories. Jogging for seven to eight hours will do it. Other activities and the calories burned for each hour spent doing them are listed in the accompanying chart.

Activity	Number of Calories Burned per Hour	Activity	Number of Calories Burned per Hour
Badminton	400	Karate	600
Baseball	350	Rowing	400
Basketball	550	Running	900
Bowling	250	Shuffleboard	250
Calisthenics	500	Skating slow	400
Croquet	250	Skating fast	600
Cycling slow	300	Skiing	450
Cycling fast	600	Soccer	650
Dancing slow	350	Softball	350
Dancing fast	600	Squash	550
Field hockey	500	Swimming slow	400
Football	600	Swimming fast	800
Golfing	250	Tennis, singles	450
Handball	550	Tennis, doubles	350
Hiking	400	Volleyball	350
Horseback riding	250	Walking slow	200
Jogging	600	Walking fast	300

Starting Tomorrow

This is the most common form of self-delusion. It is the old game of "mañana." It is self-delusion that makes the calendar seem to be your ally when in truth it is your enemy. It is also expressed as "I'll begin the day after Thanksgiving," or some other holiday, or after a visit from a relative, or the New Year, or the Ides of March. It is so easy to slide into really believing that the day after Christmas everything will be different, that you will hop out of bed a completely new person, without your old habits, compulsions, or appetites. But it is not very likely, is it?

The Cure: Admit that you are in a rut, that you lack the desire and determination to make a fresh start. Forget the calendar, and it will no longer be your enemy or your excuse. Take a deep breath, look at yourself in the mirror, and speak the magic word "Today." Then, realizing that the moment has come, make up your mind that **right now** is when your diet begins. That is the only way you can turn your cherished dream of losing weight into reality.

CHAPTER NINE

Excuses, Excuses . . .

We have already discussed the dangers of rationalization, that is, of kidding yourself that it is the pressures of daily living that make you eat more than you want. Here are some of the excuses that people frequently use, to their own detriment. Recognize any of them?

Opulence
Or "I'm Always Surrounded by Food"

There is a familiar refrain among homemakers: "If I didn't have to cook for my family, I'd have no problem." And there is the waiter who claims: "If I wasn't around food all the time I wouldn't be fat."

It would be Utopian if former alcoholics could live in a society where there was no alcohol, but, instead, they must learn to live within society as it exists. People who are overweight must also accept the fact that we are **all** surrounded by food every day of our lives. We live in a country rich with supermarkets, specialty food stores, and delicatessens. Food of all kinds—cheap food, expensive food, nourishing food, junk food—is readily available. And food is more than fuel. It is a social symbol, used to celebrate special events of all kinds, from promotions to sailings, from births to deaths. And holidays are feast days.

Also remember, however, that no matter how much we are surrounded by opulence, we do not **have** to eat what we do not **want** to eat. Slim people manage to pass up the goodies. As noted before, food and appetite are confused by people who are overweight. Hunger is the body's call for **energy**. Appetite is the body's call for **pleasure**. To the person who has not practiced some form of dietary discipline, hunger is indistinguishable from the pangs of appetite. Such persons must realize that they already have an overabundant supply of energy in the form of fat, which the body can convert to energy.

Depression
Or "I Eat When I'm Down"

Here is an excuse that is, to some degree, realistic. "Gee, Doctor, I'm feeling mighty depressed" is not a sentence to be brushed aside as nonsense. During a weight-loss program, it is not uncommon for people to become slightly depressed or "feel down." This usually occurs during the fourth or fifth week of dieting. It is a perfectly normal emotional reaction. I compare it to moving into a new home; there is always an emotional upheaval, a sadness in leaving old friends and a home where one has known happy days.

But do not use the "feeling blue" as an excuse to impede your progress. Depression is a perfectly normal reaction and a good sign in that it always follows a period of progress. The depression will last perhaps as long as a week or ten days, but it will pass. The best way to handle this temporary discomfort is to realize that you are in the process of making a trade. You're trading the temporary pleasure of excess food for the lasting pleasure of being slim and more attractive.

Illness
"Or When I'm Sick, I Overeat"

I cannot count the times people have told me such things as: "I must drink plenty of fruit juices and eat nourishing food to help cure my head cold." This normal life-occurrence (every person catches cold occasionally) is simply used as an excuse to eat. And that is all it is. There are other ways to get your quota of Vitamin C without the liability of excess calories.

It is important to analyze the kinds of "illness" people experience when they are beginning to diet. Not only do some get headaches, but they also complain of physical tiredness and lethargy. It is only natural for some people going on diets to experience traumatic symptomatology, which comes from physical and physiological adjustments to an intake of less food. It is a temporary state of discomfort, nothing more than a period of adjustment. Headaches, for example, are sometimes experienced by people as they begin to lose weight, but the pain is minor rather than acute and usually short-lived.

I find it fascinating that overweight people tend to gain weight when they become ill, whereas thin people usually lose weight when they are sick. One must guard against the temptation to exaggerate every small body ache, and use it as an excuse for needing "the strength only food can give." Of course any person with profound dysfunction should be checked professionally.

Age
"Or It Was Easier When I Was Younger"

Even comparatively young people, men and women in their late thirties, will say: "It's a lot harder to take off weight because I'm not young any more." A limp excuse. True, the body's metabolic process slows slightly with age, but this does not appreciably prevent losing weight. (I would say it is at the most a 5 percent factor in the body's ability to lose or keep off excess weight.)

In the large sense, age has nothing to do with losing weight, although, as we become older, we are less physically active. As we get older, and I am referring particularly to senior citizens and people who have retired, we also have more time on our hands. And that time, in psychological terms, weighs heavily. Because the older person feels frustrated by inactivity and lack of involvement in purposeful pursuits, he or she is driven to seek satisfaction that is, in the social sense, more isolated than previously. Or, to put it another way, one is more dependent upon deriving pleasure alone. And this seeking pleasure often takes the form of giving more attention to food.

Case History. I had always thought of my father as a thin, trim, fine example of health and manhood. My mother was roly-poly, and I'm sure I picked up my early tendency to enjoy food from her. When my father retired, he developed a bit of a paunch. He blamed it on the aging process, and swore that his intake of food had not changed. His friends all agreed that with old age comes an automatic weight gain. When he explained his plight to me, I had to disagree with his "old age" theory. The reason why my father had gained the extra weight, while maintaining the same caloric intake, was quite simple and obvious.

He had been a carpenter at a time when electric drills, saws, and other power tools were not available. During a workday he expended tremendous energy and burned up far more calories than he did in later years as a retired man. My father at first rejected this thesis, but, after consideration, agreed that the solution would be to cut his caloric intake. He did so, and is now, at eighty, a robust and slim young man.

Another reason why older people seem to have more difficulty losing weight has to do with secondary sexual feelings. But this problem is psychological, not physical. As we get older, some of us have less need to feel slender and attractive to others. Since thinness mainly depends upon this state of mind, loss of it tends to invite obesity. Re-education can help the overweight senior citizen concerning feelings of secondary sexuality.

Body Tone
"Or I'll Get Flabby If I Lose Weight"

Whether you will get flabby as you lose bulk depends on such factors as the length of time you have been heavy. The longer the time period, for instance, the greater the chance of flab. Another factor is heredity, or how flabby your mother and father were. A further consideration is the number of times you have regained lost weight. The more often this has happened, the more the skin stretches and shrinks and loses tone.

So the answer is yes and no, depending on the individual. But to be philosophical, even if you do get a little flabby, a thin and somewhat flabby body is far more attractive than a firm, fat body. (Is there such a thing?) Few people are likely to see you naked in any case. For more on body shaping, see Chapter Ten.

Appearance
"Or When I Lose Weight My Face Gets Drawn"

Nonsense, you look better. It simply takes time for you and others to become accustomed to your new appearance. But their reaction to your new thinness often acts as your excuse. As an example, when I was in professional school, I was a fat, roly-poly student. Twenty years later, and seventy-five pounds thinner, I visited my alma mater. When he saw me, the first words out of the mouth of my favorite neurology professor were: "Alex, what happened? Are you sick? Your face looks so drawn!" If he had said this years earlier, when I had first lost weight, I would have been very upset. But since it was twenty years later, I knew how to handle the situation. I knew that my one hundred pound loss was beneficial to my appearance because that fact had been confirmed countless times by other people's opinions. My former professor simply was not used to seeing me thin. I was a "new" person to him. As your face and body thin down, you become **more**, not less, attractive.

Time
"Or I Have No Time To Prepare Special 'Diet' Foods"

Even if you are not a cook, you can buy most foods of your choice already cooked or prepared, whether fresh or frozen. Do not fall victim to the myth that preparing the foods recommended in this book takes more time and labor than ordinary meal preparation. On the contrary, the foods are simple and easy to prepare and require less fussing and laboring over your stove.

Regaining Weight
"Or Why Diet? I've Always Gained It Back"

This time you are going to get thin for the correct reason. Most people initially go on diets when social pressure becomes too much to bear. This pressure is measured by a maximum weight limit that each person finds is all that he or she can emotionally accept.

Then it is time to diet and begin to lose weight. When a small amount of weight is lost, the pressure temporarily lessens. (Darling, since you lost weight you look wonderful.") With the pressure gone or lessened, the eating starts again. But this time the maximum acceptable weight level is a little higher. When this new upper level is reached, the societal pressure and the cycle begin again.

Joan came into my office forty pounds heavier than she wanted to be. Her past weight-loss history showed a spiked graph pattern that began at the age of twenty and gradually reaching higher and higher peak weights. She was disgusted with this yo-yo syndrome (fluctuating body weight). After our initial discussion, Joan realized that pressure alone would not help her keep her weight down. She learned to value her personal attractiveness, and now she is as slim as she was at the age of twenty.

Key to Happiness,
Or "When I Was Thinner, I Still Wasn't Happy"

Being thin (or fat, for that matter) does not guarantee a happy life. I know many thin people who are perfectly miserable. But being thin certainly gives you a better chance for happiness. As an example, if you should play bingo with only one card, as opposed to a friend playing with five cards, who would stand a better chance of winning? The answer is obvious.

Granted that a bingo player with only one card can win, the person with five stands a much better chance. And so it is with being thin. It does not guarantee happiness, but, over a period of time (and that is the key concept here) the chances are better. So get to it.

Tasting and Nibbling
Or "I Don't Know Why I'm Fat, I Never Overeat"

First, understand that tasting and nibbling—"noshing"—is eating. As a matter of fact, this type of insidious eating is the deadliest dietary indiscretion practiced by the overweight. It is even worse than sneak eating, because there is really no way to determine how many extra calories one takes in.

You pass the cookie jar, and so you just pinch off a small piece.

You "even off" the corners of a leftover piece of pie by eating the crumbs around it.

You steal "only a few" peanuts from the open can.

You take a swig from the open soda bottle or orange juice container or beer can.

You grab a "couple of grapes" as you pass the fruit dish.

You take a "small" spoonful of ice cream from last night's container.

You notice a leftover french fry that looks lonely while you are clearing the dinner table. So...

Those calories add up more rapidly than you may realize. The average person is not really quite aware of how many extra calories can be ingested from these tidbits.

One summer day my wife and I were invited to a friend's home to see his new pool. As we admired the construction, I noticed a very slow leak in the pool's fill spout. I asked my host why he had not had it repaired. He said he felt it was unnecessary since the very slow dripping into the pool would keep it at the proper water level, and, if there were excess water, it would simply overflow. Another guest, a plumber, heard our conversation. With a knowing smile he asked our host for a five-gallon water bucket that he placed under the leaking fill spout. To our surprise, the bucket was filled by the end of one hour. This meant that 120 gallons of water were being wasted every day. Not only was this ecologically unsound, but we estimated that it cost the pool's owner an extra sixty dollars per year for water taxes. He had the leak fixed. The person who "only nibbles" is actually eating an amazingly large quantity of food.

Handling Compliments
Or "Compliments Make Me Quit My Diet"

Compliments can be detrimental unless you learn how to deal with them. After you have lost your first ten or twelve pounds, your friends will probably tell you how wonderful you look, adding a cheery, "Keep up the good work!" You will smile and accept their kind words happily. You will probably even feel quite proud of yourself. But beware.

When complimented too often, people tend to become complacent and lose sight of their ultimate goal, but there is another reason not to take those kind words too seriously. Many people who compliment you are actually jealous of your partial success. When they say, "Keep it up," they're really thinking "She'll never do it. This is just one of those diet trips— she'll put the weight right back on again." When you have lost even more weight, the same friends will likely tell you: "You look wonderful. Don't lose another pound." At that point, be even more careful. It is true that now you look better than you ever have before, but your appearance is nothing compared to how you will look when you take off all your excess weight. Odd as it may sound, it is only when people start telling you "You look too thin" that you should begin to feel you have succeeded.

As I have explained before, it takes time for those who knew you when you were overweight to accept you as thin and normal looking. When someone compliments you while you're reducing, simply say, "Thank you," and silently rededicate yourself to losing all of the weight you want to lose and not regaining it.

The Amount of Food Consumed
Or "I Really Don't Eat Much"

It's been proven a thousand times that, five minutes after people eat, they forget having done so. If you really want to know how much you eat, simply list all the foods that you ingest for one week on the form that is shown in Illustration 5. If you are honest and keep careful and accurate count, it will be an eye opener, and you will understand full well why you are overweight.

Illustration 5
Seven-Day Honesty Report

List All Foods That You Eat and Drink

	Today	Tomorrow	3rd Day
Breakfast			
Lunch			
Dinner			
What Else?			

4th Day	5th Day	6th Day	7th Day

Small Weight Loss
Or "I'm Slightly Overweight, but I Don't Look That Bad"

People who have only from five to ten pounds of weight to lose have a problem. They really **do not** look bad, but that five or ten pounds can really be important to them.

I was delivering a lecture to a local women's club, and, at the conclusion of my talk, I called for questions. One woman asked how she could rid herself of 5 pounds that she could not lose or lost only temporarily. (Out of the corner of my eye I noticed other overweight women smiling as if to say to themselves, "I wish that were **my** problem.") I smiled wisely and replied, "Madam, you look perfectly 'OK' to me—I wouldn't worry about losing weight." The audience all grunted in agreement. The woman sat down, and the questioning resumed.

At the end of the lecture the "thin" woman approached me and said with venom, "Dr. Matos, you have no right to tell me not to lose weight. To me, my weight problem is very real and I think you were wrong to embarrass me in front of all my friends."

I promptly apologized, for she was right. To her, the five or ten pounds were just as important as twenty or thirty pounds would have been to a more obese person.

This woman was a living example of the truism that the closer you are to your goal weight, the more difficult it seems to achieve. Not only do you have to deal with your own feelings, but you must be able to shield yourself from the compliments of friends—and to stick to your diet!

The Value of Appearance
Or "I Want to be Loved for Myself, Not My Body"

Being loved for one's self is certainly a reasonable expectation. We should be judged by our capabilities and not by the size of our waists. In our society, however, it just does not work that way. Right or wrong, it is easier to arouse love initially when you are slim than when you are not.

Rapid Weight Loss and Regaining
Or "Although I Can Lose Five to Ten Pounds, in a Few Days, I Regain It More Rapidly"

You are losing and gaining water, not fat. Rapid weight gain or loss can usually be explained by transient water (fluid) that your body contains. Depending upon your weight, the amount of water can vary from zero to ten pounds. When you diet, even for a few days, your body will eliminate much of it.

That is why the weekend dieter does well for two days, jumps on the scale and is amazed at the weight loss. However, just **one** day of overeating brings back all of the water. People must be aware of this bodily mechanism if they are to lose weight successfully.

Illustration 6a

LOSS OF BODY FLUID THROUGH RAPID LOSS OF WEIGHT

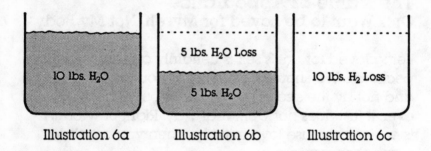

Illustration 6a   Illustration 6b   Illustration 6c

Illustration 6a—LOSS OF BODY FLUID THROUGH RAPID LOSS OF WEIGHT shows the normal amount of "losable" body water. Illustration 6b shows the water that can be lost in just two days of dieting (depending on your weight). Illustration 6c shows the amount that can be lost in four days of dieting.

CHAPTER TEN

Do-It-Yourself Aids

Thyroid Function Test

If, after reading the section on metabolism, you still believe that you are not losing weight because of an underactive thyroid, here is a simple and effective test that you can perform yourself by simply using a good fever thermometer:

- —Take your basic body temperature for three days in a row.
- —Place shaken down thermometer under your arm for ten minutes every morning **before** getting out of bed.
- —If the **average** three day reading is under 97.8 degrees, it **may** indicate an underactive or sluggish thyroid.
- —If you are menstruating, do the test from the third to the fifth day of your period.
- —Positive results should be checked professionally.

Suggest to your physician the use of kelp and Vitamin B1 if a deficiency is confirmed and found to be slight.

Spot Reducing with Manual Lipotraumatization

How many times have you lost weight only to find that the weight loss occurs in the wrong portion of your body? This frustrating experience seems to be the rule rather than the exception with most weight-loss patients.

Women, especially, complain that even after substantial weight loss, their thighs remain heavy; rather than losing the fat around the thighs, their breasts shrink. Men complain that it is difficult to get rid of the paunchy belly.

The most popular "solution" for the problem up to now has been physical exercise. But, unfortunately, exercise simply augments muscles. It does nothing to eliminate excess specific areas of fat.

The theory that governs manual lipotraumatization technique (breaking down fat by hand), is that if a "fat" area is mechanically broken down by hand, the body, while reducing via diet, will take the path of least resistance and pull or utilize or burn the fatty tissue from the area of traumatization. In other words, the body will take the path of least resistance and use the partially broken-down (traumatized) fat first. (NOTE: Do not confuse spot reducing and the technique that I am describing with treatment for cellulite, that is, small lumps or blobs of fatty deposits.)

The objective of manual lipotraumatization is to soften fatty areas so that the body, in the process of burning fat, will give priority to these problem spots. The technique is simple and consists of kneading by hand.* Since the areas of kneading do not necessarily involve the target site, I will explain how the technique applies to the most popular trouble spots, but, first, learn how to do it.

The basic technique consists of rapid kneading or squeezing by hand. Use one or both hands simultaneously. Form hands as per diagram, opposing the fingers but not the thumb (see Illustration 7).

Hand Position for Manual Lipotraumatization

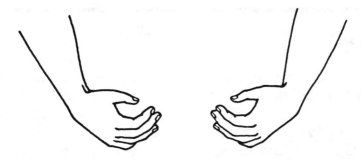

Illustration 7

Hold the fat tissue between the thumb and the fingers. Once held, roll the tissue forward and squeeze gently. Repeat this movement rapidly fifty times for each section you work on. Be careful not to squeeze too hard as you might create black-and-blue marks (hematoma). Now, here is how to work on specific trouble spots.

*NOTE: If you have varicose veins or any vascular disease, do not attempt the kneading technique.

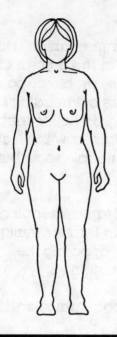 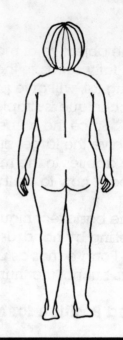

THIGHS

Do this exercise either standing or lying on your back. If you want to lose at site A, work on site B because the fatty tissue between the legs is usually looser and "mushier" than the outer aspects of the thigh. As the body utilizes the inner thigh's fatty tissue, it will tend to pull or stretch the excess tissue from the outer thigh and thus produce the desired results.

BUTTOCKS:

Do this exercise standing or lying on your stomach. To lose at site A, work on the tissue at site B if site B is looser. If it is not, then knead directly on site A.

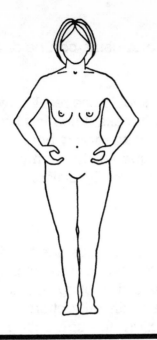

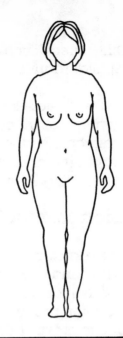

ABDOMEN:

Do this standing or lying on your back. If you wish to lose at site A, check the tissue at site B to determine which is looser. Work on the area that is looser.

BREASTS:

Although not too many women wish to lose breast size, you can use the lipotraumatization technique to "lift" the breasts. Work on site A to achieve this. As tissue is lost above the breasts, it will tend to bring the breasts up. Do not work on the breasts themselves.

Other areas, such as arms and chins, can be done in a similar manner.

Do the exercises daily. You should see results, even if only minimal, in roughly two weeks. If nothing happens, discontinue the therapy (of kneading, not dieting). Remember, this technique will help only if you are dieting. By itself, it is completely useless.

Tension Eliminator

Everyone knows that being relaxed helps one to perform any kind of work more effectively, whether physical or mental. Relaxation also aids dieting, in that tension often produces a sense of dissatisfaction, causing one to crave "false satisfaction" through eating.

The primary site of muscle tension in the human body is in the neck and shoulder areas. This body location is very important because the entire nervous system stemming from the brain is compressed into the restricted area of the neck via the spinal cord. Tense neck muscles can impinge upon this relatively unguarded area of our spinal cord and cause tension. Correct exercises eliminate this problem, for tension and relaxation cannot exist simultaneously.

Some simple neck and shoulder exercises will relax these important areas. They can be performed prior to Hypnosis II or at any other time. Perform these exercises slowly. Stretch to your full range of flexibility, but do not force to the point of discomfort.

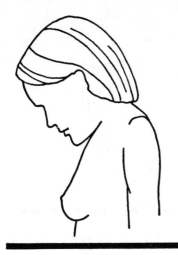

1. Bend head forward and touch chin to chest. Hold position while counting: 1 thousand, 2 thousand, 3 thousand, 4 thousand, 5 thousand. Return head to normal position.

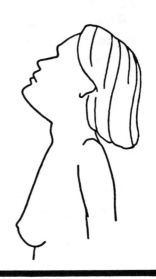

2. Bend head backward as much as possible. Hold position while counting as above. Return head to normal position.

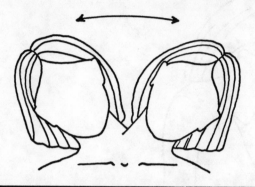

3. Bend head to the right side as much as possible and hold for the same count. Return to normal position.

4. Bend head to the left side as much as possible. Hold for the same count.

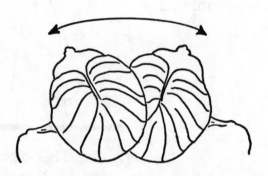

5. Rotate head to the left. Hold for the same count.

6. Rotate head to the right. Hold for the same count.

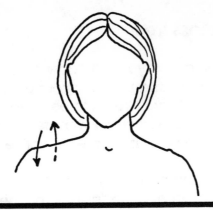

7. Elevate right shoulder
   and rotate backwards
   five times. Then for-
   ward, five times.

8. Elevate left shoulder
   and repeat.

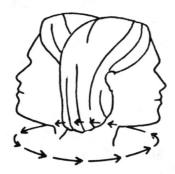

9. Rotate head in a
   circular motion, five
   times. First to the right
   and then to the left.

That is it. This entire procedure should take no more
than three minutes.

Attractiveness Test

Have you ever asked yourself, "How attractive am I?" I'm sure you have, and perhaps your answer was not what you would have liked it to be. The truth of the matter is that, as attractive as you are presently, by being thinner you can be **more** attractive.

I have devised a simple test to illustrate numerically just exactly where one "stands" on the attractiveness spectrum. I call it the physical attractiveness or PA Factor. It is calculated by using numerical percentages of from 1 to 100. Each percentage point represents one pound of weight. Ideally, individuals who are content with their present weight would possess the highest possible PA Factor of 100 percent. A person who expresses the desire to lose ten pounds would have a PA Factor of 90 percent. A wish to lose twenty pounds would mean a rate of 80 percent, and so forth. The thinner one is, the higher the score.

Use this test and remember your starting PA Factor percentage. Although there are no passing or failing scores, you will remain on your diet until your PA Factor is 100 percent.

Image Visualization

Did you ever wonder how you would look if you lost all of the weight you wanted to lose? With this in mind, a manufacturer created a "magic" mirror which could be adjusted to show how the overweight individual would look after losing five, ten, and twenty or more pounds. He felt that, by seeing themselves thin, fat people would be able to visualize the end result of dieting and thus be inspired to their goal weight. Unfortunately, the mirror is very expensive and beyond the means of most people, but there is a simple, inerxpensive device that achieves the same end. Simply paste a picture of your head, taken from an old photo, upon the body of the picture of a thin person. Hold it at arms length and smile. This is the future "you."

Behavior Modification

When Pavlov's dog began to salivate at the tinkling of a bell, **behavior modification** was born. A bell was rung, and the dog was fed. After a while, the animal associated the ringing bell with food and would salivate automatically when it was rung, even without the presence of food. Overweight people do the same thing when they associate eating with a certain circumstance and surrounding.

The idea behind behavior modification is to change these external "clues" that are associated with food, thereby making dieting easier. Here are the basic principles.

1 **Eat slowly.**
   —Slow eating tends to satisfy more.
   —Eat soup with a teaspoon.
   —Do not eat while reading, watching television, or talking on the telephone.
   —Pay attention to your food and receive the maximum enjoyment from it.
   —Take small bites and chew thoroughly.

2 **Eat at the same location.**
   —When home, eat in the kitchen or dining room only.
   —Avoid your favorite easy chair where many prior dietary discretions probably took place.

3. **Sit down to eat.**
   —Never eat while standing, especially if you should be near the refrigerator or a pantry or talking on the telephone.

4. **Eat from a small plate.**
   —This tends to make your portions seem larger.

5. **Eating out.**
   —Never look at a menu since you know what you should eat.
   —Avoid ethnic restaurants, especially Chinese and Italian ones.
   —Do not arrive at the restaurant earlier than necessary.
   —Do not linger later than necessary.
   —Avoid restaurants that serve "family" style.

6. **Shopping for food.**
   —Shop **after** eating.
   —Shop with a prepared list.
   —Don't "window shop" at the supermarket.

7. **Do not become obsessed with dieting.**
   —Make it a part of your everyday existence, like brushing your teeth.

CHAPTER ELEVEN

Living Within Your Seams

The Plateau: Getting "Stuck"

I have encountered many people like Louise, whose starting weight was 175 pounds and whose goal weight was 130 pounds. She lost 30 pounds without any great struggle, but remained at 145 pounds for over a month. Quite naturally, she could not understand why, and she was disappointed.

The answer to such a problem is simple. If "plateauing" lasts longer than a month, one of two things is usually happening. For one thing, the person may be gradually adding foods in small amounts. The amount of food may not be enough to cause weight gain, but it can slow weight loss. If the extra eating continues, there is no further weight loss, and the would-be dieter gets "stuck." The second possibility is that often people such as Louise never really adhere to the Apple Diet. They do eat less than usual, and so the effect is to lose a certain amount and then get stuck at a plateau. The person may accept the principles of my diet, but does not follow it to the letter and, thereby, consumes too many calories to allow continued weight loss. You cannot combine diets. You must stick to one diet at a time to be successful.

Maintenance Made Easy

Understanding Deficit Eating

Recidivism (regaining lost weight) is the dieter's greatest pitfall. Without exception, every dieter I treat emphatically says: "Once I take off this weight, I'll never put it back on again. Wouldn't I be silly to exert effort, time, and money to lose and then get fat again?" And yet, sadly, many patients do. They unconsciously look forward to getting thin so that they can eat again.

Deficit eating is an important concept that must be clearly understood by new "thin" people. They can never eat as they did when they were overweight, and they must often eat **less** food than will sustain their goal weight. There is a reason for this. It means that occasional overeating will not then add unwanted pounds. The truth of the matter is that, even when you have become thin, you must remain on the partial diet because, to the overweight person, "normal" eating means overeating.

Steps for Remaining Thin

Once a person reaches the goal weight, I allow sensible deviation from the formal structure of total dieting. I call my method the "Two in Seven Plan." Proceed as follows: Diet for five days and allow extra eating for two. The two nondieting days can be bunched together or kept separate. (For example, they can be Monday and Thursday, or, if you prefer, a weekend.) Do not let your weight fluctuate by more than three pounds. Although you can never eat the way you did before, you can keep off the weight lost for the rest of your life if your planned eating indiscretions are reasonable and controlled.

A Final Word

Once you have lost all of your excess weight, you will have established proper eating habits. You will also have gained the deep subconscious desire to be as attractive as possible by remaining thin. Having gained greater self-respect, you will be able to live life more fully and to enjoy yourself more. Your personality and talents will bloom, and you will feel free to show, and to be, the person you truly are.

And you can do that.

CHAPTER TWELVE
Diet Profile Questionnaire

Each of us is unique, and our weight problems vary. There are degrees of "fatness" and "thinness." However, to fit the context of this questionnaire, I stick to the definitions of fat and thin used earlier. A fat person is defined as one who is not satisfied with his or her weight and desires to lose, while a thin person is satisfied with his or her present weight. I'm talking about **conditionally**, rather than genetically, thin people. In other words, about thin people who have had to reduce or watch their weight (as opposed to naturally thin people who never have such a problem; see Chapter Two).

Over a period of five years, I have presented this questionnaire to 250 fat and 250 thin people chosen from my patient roster. Their average age was about thirty, and they were slightly above average income. Sixty percent were female. None of the overweight group inquired as to why they were being asked to complete the questionnaire. (They probably assumed it to be a necessary component of their therapy.) But most members of the thin group did express curiosity. After a brief explanation, all in the thin group eagerly cooperated.

The questionnaire was composed of thirty-nine questions, which were designed to offer a graphic picture of the motives and attitudes, the strengths and weaknesses, of overweight as opposed to thin people. Following the questionnaire, the answers are analyzed. Before studying such statistics, however, write out your own answers so you can compare them to those given by the people questioned. By so doing you can learn exactly how "fat" or "thin" your own thinking turns out to be.

THE QUESTIONS

Check one blank space as an answer to each question, unless otherwise indicated:

1. How is your general physical health?

   a. good ( )
   b. fair ( )
   c. poor ( )

2. How is your general mental health?

   a. good ( )
   b. fair ( )
   c. poor ( )

3. How intelligent do you consider yourself?

   a. above average ( )
   b. average ( )
   c. below average ( )

4. How sexually attractive do you consider yourself?

   a. above average ( )
   b. average ( )
   c. below average ( )

5. Were you overweight as a child (pre teenager)?

   yes ( )
   no ( )

6. Were you overweight as a teenager?

yes ( )
no ( )

7. When you were a child, was your mother overweight?

yes ( )
no ( )

8. When you were a child, was your father overweight?

yes ( )
no ( )

9. Do you have any brothers or sisters who are now overweight?

yes ( )
no ( )

10. Were your parents weight conscious?

yes ( )
no ( )

11. Do you eat three "regular" meals a day?

yes ( )
no ( )

12. Do you eat between-meal snacks?

      yes ( )
      no   ( )

13. Do you eat a nutritionally balanced diet?

      yes ( )
      no   ( )

14. Do you eat breakfast?

      yes ( )
      no   ( )

15. On a yearly average, how many pounds do you fluctuate?

    a.   0- 5   ( )
    b.   5-10   ( )
    c.   10-20   ( )
    d.   20 and above ( )

16. When dieting, how often do you weigh yourself?

    a.   daily (or more) ( )
    b.   weekly   ( )
    c.   bimonthly   ( )
    d.   monthly   ( )
    e.   rarely   ( )

17. When **not** dieting, how often do you weigh yourself?

  a. daily or more) ( )
  b. weekly   ( )
  c. bimonthly   ( )
  d. monthly   ( )
  e. rarely   ( )

18. Do you dine out often (dinner only)?

  yes ( )
  no ( )

19. Do you have regular eating time periods?

  yes ( )
  no ( )

20. Are you constantly seeking a "good diet" to help you lose or maintain your weight?

  yes ( )
  no ( )

21. Have you ever taken diet pills in order to lose weight?

  yes ( )
  no ( )

22. If the answer to the above is yes, did you lose weight with the pills?

       yes   ( )
       no   ( )

23. Are you aware that taking pills can be addictive and detrimental to your health?

       yes   ( )
       no   ( )

24. Do you believe that you have little or no will-power when it comes to food?

       yes   ( )
       no   ( )

25. Do you believe that losing weight or keeping thin is more difficult for you than it is for others?

       yes   ( )
       no   ( )

26. Do you find that if you keep busy, it's easier to eat less?

       yes   ( )
       no   ( )

27. During happy times do you eat—

       a.   less   ( )
       b.   the same   ( )
       c.   more   ( )

28. During unhappy times do you eat—

    a.   less   ( )
    b.   the same   ( )
    c.   more   ( )

29. During which time period do you find it most difficult to control your appetite?

    a.   morning   ( )
    b.   afternoon   ( )
    c.   evening   ( )

30. Do you wake up during the night to eat?

    yes   ( )
    no   ( )

31. Which of the following food groups appeals to you most?

    a.   sweets   ( )
    b.   starches   ( )
    c.   proteins, meats, eggs, etc. ( )
    d.   vegetables   ( )
    e.   alcoholic beverages   ( )

32. Do you feel guilty after eating foods that will tend to make you gain weight?

    yes   ( )
    no   ( )

33. When deciding what to eat for a meal, are you consciously aware of the caloric value of these foods?

>   yes ( )
>   no ( )

34. Do you believe that eating wisely is a habit that can be cultivated?

>   yes ( )
>   no ( )

35. In your opinion, your present weight is due primarily to which of the following?

>   a.   hereditary factors   ( )
>   b.   environmental factors   ( )
>   c.   conscious control   ( )
>   d.   keeping physically active   ( )
>   e.   other   ( )

Explain:

36. Why (for thin people) do you stay thin or (for fat people) want to be thin?

CHECK ONE OR MORE
>   a.   for health reasons: less chance of developing heart disease, diabetes, etc.   ( )
>   b.   to feel physically better and have more energy   ( )
>   c.   for advancement in the business world   ( )
>   d.   to look better in clothes   ( )

e.	to be attractive	( )
f.	to satisfy my spouse	( )
g.	to provide a good example	( )
h.	for my children	( )
i.	other	( )

Explain:

37. If you have checked more than one choice in the above question, which do you consider the most important?

a.	( )
b.	( )
c.	( )
d.	( )
e.	( )
f.	( )
g.	( )
h.	( )
i.	( )

38. For a generous payment, would you take part in an experiment which would necessitate your gaining 20 percent more poundage than your present body weight, and keeping that extra weight on for six months?

yes	( )
no	( )

39. If your answer to the above is no, please check the most important reason why.

a. afraid you'd never be able to lose the weight ( )

b. afraid the "eating more" habit would be hard to break ( )

c. danger to your health ( )

d. being less attractive ( )

Related Statistics

A study of the following statistics will demonstrate clear differences in the general pattern of thought and attitudes of fat and thin people. It will also give you a personal "diet profile" by letting you see how your own answers measure up against those of the thousand people questioned.

1. Physical health—Of the thin people, 89 percent, compared to 76 percent of the overweight, considered themselves to be in good health. This percent remained the same for the fair and poor health categories. The obvious conclusion is that fat people suffer more physical ills than thin people, a point I established in Chapter Two.

2. Mental health—This question was intended to obtain very general subjective feelings about how the two groups viewed their state of happiness

		Percentage of Groups	
		FAT	THIN
a.	good	85	93
b.	fair	13	6
c.	poor	2	1

Overweight people seem to suffer more stress than thin people.

3. Intelligence—This category was created to discover how "smart" our subjects considered themselves. Every person has a "gut" feeling about his intelligence. Whatever our physical limitations, we all have the ability to weigh and measure, to think and understand. Both groups fared the same. This would seem to indicate that intelligence, or belief of intelligence, has nothing to do with being fat or thin.

4. Sexual Attractiveness—From the results of this question it becomes obvious that one's estimate of personal appeal to the opposite sex is directly related to being thin or fat:

		Percentage of Group	
		FAT	THIN
a.	above	2	33
b.	above	24	63
c.	below	54	4

Here we have a clear picture of inferiority feelings and low self-esteem.

5, 6, 7, 8, 9, and 10. History of being overweight—Since this category is broken down into numerous questions, we can recognize a general trend by studying the results: Of all the overweight people questioned. 21 percent were overweight as preteen children; 45 percent as teenagers. Of the thin group, 18 percent were overweight as preteenagers; only 8 percent as teenagers. (They were beginning to cope with their problem.) Of the overweight group, 78 percent had an overweight father or mother; 20 percent had two overweight parents. Of the thin people, on a comparative basis, 40 percent had one overweight parent; 11 percent had two overweight parents. Of the fat people, 23 percent claimed that one or both of their parents were weight conscious; of the thin people, 57 percent claimed one or both of their parents were weight conscious. This last statistic I find fascinating. It proves that thin parents are more conscious of slim bodies as representing an ideal than fat parents. Therefore, the training, education, and even the food that the children of thin parents receive (as well, of course, as their eating habits) differ from the influences overweight parents exert on their offspring.

11, 12, and 13. Regularity of eating habits—Again, the questions here can be broken down into simple conclusions: Only 26 percent of overweight people stick to three regular meals a day, as compared to 67 percent of thin people. Over 78 percent of the overweight eat between-meal snacks, while only 12 percent of thin people indulge in this habit.

(**Note:** this does not include the coffee break, which would markedly increase the percentages in both categories. But statistics concerning the coffee break would not be truly indicative; the chances are that the overweight eat more. Of the fat 18 percent, versus 31 percent of the thin, eat a nutritionally balanced diet.

14. Eating Breakfast—This category dramatically differentiates the groups. Only 10 percent of the overweight people eat breakfast, compared to 89 percent of the thin group. As I pointed out, the first group skips breakfast because "I have no time to eat breakfast," or, "I'm not hungry." Actually, such people are giving themselves an excuse to overeat at a later time because "after all, I skipped breakfast, so I have it coming to me."

15. Weight Fluctuation—Of the thin people, 92 percent held their weight at plus or minus five pounds. Of the fat group, 2 percent fluctuated from zero to five pounds, 8 percent from five to ten pounds, 32 percent from ten to twenty pounds and 58 percent from twenty pounds and above per year. Why? Because they stumble from one diet to another in a desperate attempt to find one that will satisfy their appetite, rather than understanding the true nature of their problem.

16 and 17. Weighing—When dieting, the fat people weighed themselves on an average of five times a week. When not dieting, they rarely weighed in. Thin people weighed themselves on an average of once a week, whether or not they were dieting. Obviously, the fat person's erratic use of the scale does not aid in taking off weight (see Chapter Five).

18. Frequency of dining out—Both groups fared the same in this area. This fact negates two popular excuses: "If I didn't eat out so much, I could be more in control of my appetite," and "If I could only get out of the kitchen, I'd eat less."

19. Regular eating—time periods—Of those who are overweight, 92 percent said they did not have regular times to eat. They eat on impulse, because of a sudden rush of appetite or some mental image. Of the thin group, 71 percent had regular times to eat. This shows that thin people have structured time periods and eat because of physiological (physical) need rather than psychological (mental) fulfillment.

20. Seeking a good diet—Of the overweight, 99 percent were seeking one. Most said they had tried at least eight diets. Only 18 percent of the thin group admitted to seeking a "good diet" constantly. The remaining 82 percent of the thin group explained that it was not necessary for them to seek new diets because they knew that eating less food would keep them thin. This fact, therefore, is known to both groups. It is obvious that thin people use correct thinking in addition to proper diet as a fundamental device to remain thin. They do not depend on the hope for a miracle diet.

21, 22, and 23. Using diet pills—Of the overweight, 88 percent had tried diet pills; 38 percent of the thin people. Of those who used them, 89 percent lost weight. Over 98 percent reported that their weight loss was temporary. In both groups, 98 percent of the overweight and 93 percent of the thin people realized that diets pills can be addictive and detrimental to health.

24 and 25. Willpower and ability for thinness—Here again the overweight respondents scored "low": 94 percent as compared to 18 percent. It is **motivation** that must be cultivated if one is to lose weight, not "willpower." Of the overweight group, 98 percent said that it is difficult to lose or keep off weight, as compared to 62 percent of the thin group. And yet, the thin people keep thin because they are truly motivated to do so.

26. Eating as related to keeping busy—Of the thin people, 84 percent said that the factor of how busy they were was not related to eating. The views of the overweight were completely opposite in that 94 percent said that keeping busy helped keep their mind off food. (Remember, the thin people said that it did not matter.) Since it is impossible to keep busy at all times, one is constantly facing opportunities to eat. Idle time is as "normal" as being occupied. One cannot be constantly busy.

27 and 28. Emotional eating—Emotions carried little weight with thin people. During happy or unhappy times their diet did not vary. With the others, however, it was quite a different story, for 82 percent said they eat the same or more when they are happy (for example, "I got married and became content") and 86 percent said they eat the same or more when they are unhappy (for example, "The kids get on my nerves"). This statistic more than proves how the normal state of affairs is used as another excuse for dietary indiscretions. After all, happiness and unhappiness are normal.

29. Controlling the appetite by time periods—Thin people found no difference among the three time periods. Among the others, 3 percent found it hardest to control their appetites in the morning, 16 percent in the afternoon, and 81 percent in the evening. I believe evening is the major problem simply because people have finished work and are free to do as they please. This applies to weekends, vacations, and other free times.

30. Waking up during the night to eat—Only 1 percent of the thin people answered affirmatively, and most explained that at such times they ate only because they were awake and eating took place only when they occasionally slept poorly, at which point they had a light snack. The other answers were quite different. Only 2 percent admitted to eating at night, but they did so on a regular basis, that is, every night (for more on night eating, see Chapter Four).

31. Appeal of food groups—Thin people answered as follows: 72 percent placed equal emphasis on proteins, fruits, and vegetables; 9 percent on alcoholic beverages, and 19 percent on sweets and starches. Of the overweight group, 47 percent admitted a preference for sweets; 32 percent for starches; 12 percent for proteins; 3 percent for fruits and vegetables, and only 1 percent for alcoholic beverages.

32. Guilt from eating fattening foods—Over 92 percent of the thin people said they felt no guilt. They reasoned that, if they feasted heavily during a holiday or special occasion, it would do no harm and add no extra weight. But 98 percent of the overweight group felt guilt. Obviously guilt is not a deterrent to overeating.

33. Conscious awareness of the caloric value of foods—Almost all of the people questioned (92 percent) were aware of the caloric value of foods, but the thin group had only a general idea of calories. They knew, for example, that there were many calories in a piece of pie and few in spinach. The average overweight person, on the contrary, could probably tell you the caloric value of a grape pit, but this knowledge, by itself, does not seem to cut down the total food intake. It just adds to the guilt.

34. The wisdom of cultivating good eating habits—This is the only question on which all people in both groups agreed. Everyone felt it was wise to cultivate good eating habits. Then why don't more people do it? For all of the reasons given in this book.

35. The primary cause of present body weight—Of the five categories of choice, 32 percent of the overweight blamed their weight on "hereditary factors," 28 percent on environmental factors, and 72 percent on a combination of both factors. Only 8 percent admitted that the factor of "conscious control" played a role, and only 21 percent admitted the importance of "keeping physically active." Among the thin people, the most meaningful statistic was that 78 percent felt that both "hereditary" and "environmental" factors were important, but that these were not the only reasons for their trim bodies. As many as 87 percent believed that "keeping physically active" and "conscious control" were also factors. In short, the large majority of those who are overweight tended to blame heredity and environment and to minimize the importance of their own eating habits and lack of personal pride.

36 and 37. Wanting to become or stay thin—
Among the thin people, less than 9 percent were influenced by only a single reason, while 91 percent felt that all of the reasons were valid. But when pressed to name the most important factor, most emphasis (79 percent was for "looking better in clothes," and "being more attractive." After that, the thin people chose, in this order b, a, f, g and c. Among the fat group, few who chose only one category, for 86 percent felt that all seven reasons were important. When pressed for the most important factor, however, the greatest emphasis was placed upon "health" (52 percent), and "to feel physically better and have more energy" (27 percent). In the **combined** categories of "clothes" and "attractive," the overweight only scored 10 percent. I found it interesting to note that these responses were totally the reverse of the thin answers. Although all of the categories in this question are

sound and inspirational, obviously only a few really work. To become thin, those who are overweight must learn to revamp their thinking.

38 and 39. Willingness to participate in the experiment for pay—Thin people seemed terrified by the proposition, since only 2 percent would have put on the extra twenty pounds for six months. It seems that they guard their "thinness" as if it were Fort Knox. Of the others, 32 percent would have participated. Of those who refused, 92 percent were concerned with "being less attractive," and "afraid the 'eating more habit,'" would be hard to break. In the overweight group, only 16 percent chose those two reasons, again illustrating that thin and fat people do not think alike. The thin person considers the problem from a societal objective standpoint (how he would appear to the world), while the overweight person's concern is a very personal matter (body and weight).

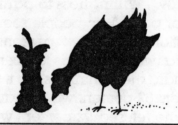

CHAPTER THIRTEEN
Mostly Chicken
By Bernice Matos

Since chicken is the mainstay of the Big Applie Diet, I have developed a variety of interesting low-calorie recipes you may want to try. I have found chicken to be a wonderful, versatile food whose taste, color, and shape can be changed with little effort. There are five classifications of this relatively inexpensive and readily available food: roasters or bakers, broilers, fryers, stewing chicken and fowl, and capons.

- **—Roasting** or **Baking Chickens** are plump and do not dry out if you cook them a little too long. I like to use roasters for my potting recipes, too.

- **—Fryers** and **Broilers** are especially good when you are in a hurry. The meat is closer to the bone and cooks faster.

—Stewing Chickens and **Fowl** are generally used for soup. The meat is usually firmer and can withstand the long cooking process without falling apart.

—Capons are chickens that have been castrated prior to puberty. This seems to increase their size and tenderness.

Choose whatever type of chicken you prefer, but I suggest the younger birds as they contain less fat and are more tender. Most chickens purchased today are ready for cooking, and you can purchase either fresh or frozen chicken whole, half, quartered, or in packages containing your favorite pieces.

Ready—to-eat chicken is also available in most parts of the country. Barbecued chicken (cooked in the store) is ideal for those who do not want to prepare their own meals, but TV dinners should be used only in emergencies as the chicken is frequently fried and breaded.

I find that when you roast a whole chicken or broil it on a rotisserie you get a juicier, more flavorful result. A whole chicken usually cooks in about an hour and a half at 325 degrees, while a cut-up chicken takes only three-quarters of an hour. Remember that stoves vary. You must judge the "doneness" according to your own stove and preference. A thermometer is helpful. Insert the thermometer into the thickest part of the chicken. When it reads 190 degrees, it is done. When baking or sauteing, remove all skin and fat **before** cooking. When broiling, remove the skin **after** cooking.

The recipes that follow are for two to four people using a two-pound chicken. If you want to prepare for a larger number of people, or to prepare food in advance, simply use multiples of all the ingredients.

EASY BASIC CHICKEN

A simple method of preparing chicken that is quick and good!

4 chicken breasts (or thighs if you prefer dark meat)

Sprinkle seasoned salt over chicken.
Broil uncovered for about ½ hour at 400°.
Do not turn.
When done, remove skin.

CHICKEN QUICK

For busy people who want to eat and get on with it.

>   4 chicken breasts
>   4 teaspoons soy sauce
>   1 tablespoon sauteed onion flakes
>   1/4 teaspoon each of garlic flakes, parsley,
>   celery
>   Dash of dill

Sprinkle herbs and seasonings lightly over chicken.
Sprinkle 1 teaspoon soy sauce over each breast.
Bake at 375° about 3/4 hour, or broil until brown.
Do not cover.
When done, remove skin.

LEMON CHICKEN

A delicate lemony tang to this one.

    4 chicken quarters
    4 tablespoons lemon juice
    1/8 teaspoon pepper
    1 teaspoon salt

Sprinkle 1/16 teaspoon pepper, 2 tablespoons lemon
juice, and 1/2 teaspoon salt over chicken.
Place chicken skin side down and broil for 10
minutes.
Turn chicken skin side up.
Season with remaining ingredients, salt, pepper, and
one tablespoon lemon juice.
Broil for 15 minutes more.
Sprinkle remaining lemon juice over chicken and
serve.

CHICKEN IN THE POT

One of the great classic chicken dishes.

  4 chicken quarters
  6 cups water
  2 medium stalks celery, chopped
  4 carrots
  1 bouillon cube
  onion, cubed

Remove all fat and skin from chicken **before**
cooking.
Cook all ingredients together for 3 hours on low heat.
It is best to prepare this one the day before, cool in
the refrigerator overnight, and then skim off all con-
gealed fat. Then simply heat and eat.

CHINESE-STYLE CHICKEN

An easy, satisfying "Chinese" dinner.

4 chicken breasts
1 cup onion wedges
1/2 cup soy sauce
1/2 teaspoon oil
1 small can bamboo shoots, drained
2 tablespoons cold water

Brown chicken in hot oil.
Add onion, bamboo shoots, soy sauce, and water.
Simmer until chicken is tender, about 3/4 hour, on low heat.
Stir occasionally to prevent sticking and scorching.

CHICKEN ITALIANO

Neither oily nor greasy—just lots of flavor!

    4 chicken quarters
    4 tablespoons low-calorie Italian dressing
    1 onion, chopped
    1/2 cup water
    1/4 teaspoon garlic powder

Combine Italian dressing with water.
Marinate chicken in mixture.
Sprinkle garlic powder over chicken.
Spread onion pieces on top of chicken.
Bake uncovered, until tender, at 375° (about 3/4 hour).

CHICKEN FRANCAIS

The French version—and very good, too!

4 chicken breasts
4 tablespoons French dressing
1 tablespoon minced or chopped onion flakes
1/2 cup water

Combine water with French dressing.
Marinate chicken breasts in mixture of dressing and water.
Sprinkle minced or chopped onion flakes over chicken.
Bake at 375°, uncovered, for about 3/4 hour.

KENTUCKY MOUNTAIN CHICKEN

Delicious—and far better for your diet than Kentucky-fried!

> 4 chicken breasts
> 1 tablespoon onion flakes
> 1 large green pepper, sliced thin
> ½ cup apple vinegar
> ½ teaspoon minced garlic

Marinate chicken breasts in vinegar.
Add spice.
Lay slices of green pepper over chicken.
Put just enough water to cover bottom of pan.
Cover and cook at 325° for about 1½ hours.

CHICKEN OREGANO

Spicy, fragrant, aromatic.

>   4 chicken breasts
>   ¼ teaspoon oregano
>   1 large onion, chopped
>   1 green pepper, chopped
>   1 small can tomato juice

Brown chicken on low heat.
Sprinkle chicken with oregano.
Scatter onion and pepper pieces over chicken.
Pour tomato juice over.
Bake, covered, in oven at 375° till done—about 1 hour.

CHICKEN BERNICE

This is one of my favorite recipes. As you will see, I combine all of my favorite ingredients, and the result is very tasty.

    4 chicken breasts
    1 tablespoon onion, minced
    1 tablespoon parsley
    1 teaspoon salt
    ¼ teaspoon garlic
    4 or 5 tablespoons soy sauce
    1 large onion, sliced thin
    1 large green pepper, sliced thin

Brown chicken on low heat in stainless steel or Teflon pan.
Sprinkle all seasoning over chicken.
Sprinkle soy sauce over each breast.
Steam onion slices until tender and put on top of chicken.
Place green pepper slices over onion slices.
Add just enough water to cover bottom of pan.
Cover and simmer 1 hour or until done to your taste.

CHICKEN AND WINE

Cuisine minceur—haute cuisine without the calories.

   4 chicken breasts
   3 tablespoons parsley
   4 tablespoons soy sauce
   2 cloves garlic, chopped
   1 large onion
   1 small can mushrooms
   ⅓ cup white cooking wine

Saute chicken until brown in Teflon pan on low heat.
Add parsley and soy sauce.
Put into baking dish.
In a separate pan, brown garlic, onions, and
mushrooms, and place over chicken.
Pour wine over chicken and bake at 350° for 1½
hours.

Note: Red or white wine is permissible, but white is
preferred as it does not change the color of the
chicken.

CHICKEN PAPRIKA

Mildly spiced Hungarian favorite.

> 4 chicken quarters
> ¼ teaspoon garlic powder
> ½ teaspoon paprika
> 4 tablespoons tomato juice

Season chicken with garlic powder and paprika.
Pour 1 tablespoon juice over each quarter.
Broil at low temperature until done (about ¾ hour).
Do not turn.

CORNISH HENS

A wonderful meal for a holiday or special occasion.

    2 cornish hens
    ½ cup vinegar, any kind, divided into 3 parts
    2 teaspoons onion, minced
    ½ tablespoon garlic powder

Baste hens with ⅓ of vinegar.
Sprinkle minced onion pieces and garlic powder on hens.
Roast in oven at 325° about 1 hour, basting at 20-minute intervals with remaining vinegar.

Note: Hens taste best if cooked very well. Outside of chicken should be well browned.

ORANGE FRUIT CHICKEN

A delightful light meal for warm weather.

4 chicken breasts
⅛ teaspoon garlic powder
½ teaspoon salt
Juice from 1 orange
1 orange, sliced thin

Marinate chicken in orange juice.
Season chicken with garlic powder and salt.
Arrange chicken in baking pan and place slices of orange around chicken.
Bake at 375° about ¾ hour (longer if you like chicken well done).

Tips . . .

To be lowest in calories, chickens should have all skin and fat removed before cooking. This, of course, tends to make the chicken a little dry, but cooking at low temperatures will help retain the moistness. If you must leave the skin on, be sure to remove it before eating.

Suggested seasonings may be replaced with seasonings of your choice. Do not be afraid to experiment. You will be surprised how different each recipe will taste when you substitute new seasonings.

Recommended natural seasonings are: celery, sea greens, mushrooms, soy bean, dill, onion, parsley, beet fructose, white pepper.

Cheese Dish

BAGEL AU GRATIN

This is one of my personal favorites for breakfast or lunch.

> Simply toast ½ bagel (a half bagel is counted as one slice of bread), spread it lightly with diet margarine, place one ounce of Muenster cheese on top, and melt in broiler.

Eat steaming hot, right out of the oven. Use a knife and fork, and cut into bite-sized pieces. This makes a delicious and extremely filling breakfast or lunch.

If you enjoy fast foods, simply prepare your cheese by using one slice of any hard cheese. Serve on a slice of bread or half a bagel. You may use pre-sliced or packaged American, Swiss, Muenster or a wedge of Gruyere. Avoid processed cheeses.